DYING: A SOCIAL PERSPECTIVE ON THE END OF LIFE

*For Sarah*

# Dying: A Social Perspective on the End of Life

ALEX BROOM
*University of New South Wales, Sydney, Australia*

Routledge
Taylor & Francis Group
LONDON AND NEW YORK

First published 2015 by Ashgate Publishing

Published 2016 by Routledge
2 Park Square, Milton Park, Abingdon, Oxon OX14 4RN
711 Third Avenue, New York, NY 10017, USA

First issued in paperback 2017

*Routledge is an imprint of the Taylor & Francis Group, an informa business*



**British Library Cataloguing in Publication Data**
A catalogue record for this book is available from the British Library.

**The Library of Congress has cataloged the printed edition as follows:**
Broom, Alex.
Dying : a social perspective on the end of life / by Alex Broom.
pages cm
Includes bibliographical references and index.
ISBN 978-1-4094-5373-4 (hardback)
1. Death – Social aspects. 2. Death – Psychological aspects. 3. Bereavement. I. Title.

HQ1073.B76 2015
306.9–dc23

ISBN 13: 978-1-138-49485-5 (pbk)
ISBN 13: 978-1-4094-5373-4 (hbk)

# Contents

# List of Abbreviations

| | |
|---|---|
| AMA | Australian Medical Association |
| BMA | British Medical Association |
| CAM | Complementary and Alternative Medicine |
| CPG | Clinical Practice Guidelines |
| EBHC | Evidence based healthcare |
| EBM | Evidence based medicine |
| EBP | Evidence based practice |
| GP | General Practitioner |
| NHS | National Health Service |
| WHO | World Health Organization |
| YIMP | Years in medical practice |

# Acknowledgements

This book was supported by funding from the Australian Research Council (ARC), namely, an ARC Future Fellowship (FT100100294) and an ARC Linkage Grant (LP120200268). Without this funding the writing of this book would not have been possible. I acknowledge the support of Assa Doron and Damien Ridge in commenting on various chapter drafts. Thanks to Suvena Sethi, for your constant support throughout the entire process of writing the manuscript. I'd like to thank Sarah, Jen, Alison and Brian for being lifelong sources of encouragement and support. Colleagues who contributed significantly to the broader program of research, which I often draw on implicitly or explicitly in this book, include Emma Kirby, Jon Adams, Phillip Good and Julia Wootton, Janet Hardy and Patsy Yates. Finally, to the participants in the studies I draw on here, I thank you once again for giving your valuable (and often limited) time to assist in developing the ideas presented in the following pages.

I note that some parts of particular chapters in this book draw from previously published material and thus the following acknowledges these works. Parts of Chapter 2 were originally published in *Social Science & Medicine*, 2013, 78(1): 9–16, DOI: 10.1016/j.socscimed.2012.11.008. Parts of Chapter 3 were originally published in *Health*, 2011, 15(1): 96–111, DOI: 10.1177/1363459309360797. Parts of Chapter 4 were originally published in *Qualitative Health Research*, 2012, 22(2): 226–37, DOI: 10.1177/1049732311421181. Parts of Chapter 5 were originally published in the *Sociology of Health and Illness*, 2013, 35(4): 499–513. DOI: 10.1111/j.1467-9566.2012.01497.x. Parts of Chapter 6 were originally published in *Qualitative Health Research*, 2014, DOI: 1049732314553123. Parts of Chapter 8 were originally published in *Social Science & Medicine*, 2010, 71(5): 869–76. DOI: 10.1016/j.socscimed.2010.05.026.

# Chapter 1
# Introduction

The usual response from colleagues when I mentioned I was writing a book on dying was to hurry the conversation on to another matter. Who could blame them? To say dying is not a sexy issue in the West is an understatement, especially dying of a disease like cancer. In writing this book, I discovered that dying continues to be shunned as a legitimate topic in polite circles, despite its ubiquity. If it is mentioned, then it is all too easily dispensed with, with a joke perhaps. No doubt for most of us death conjures up strong feelings at some level. We project all kinds of fears onto it. After all, the topic of death can trigger strong feelings of grief, sympathy and introspection. However, there are cracks in this story. For instance, 'heroic' deaths (Seale 1995) might receive sustained media attention, dinner party chatter and prolonged memorialisation that 'everyday' varieties of death and dying do not. While there has been some erosion of cultural taboos around death and dying in recent years (Lee 2008; Sayer 2010; Willmott 2000), dying is still often resisted, ignored, stigmatised, laughed away, pushed aside or otherwise cloaked in shadows. I venture that these perceptions and responses position dying as a pivotal moment for contemporary sociological inquiry.

Dying conjures up the most difficult and confronting of all experiences we can imagine in the West. With this in mind, it is entirely understandable that death has received relatively limited attention in the public sphere or indeed within the scholarly literature prior to mid-to-late twentieth century (e.g. Faunce and Fulton 1958; Glaser and Strauss 1968). It represents the end of our embodied connection with the world. Death is the final democratic process we enter, and we all eventually experience it, involving as it surely must, the fracture of our remaining social ties. This critical social occasion, not only affects the dying but also profoundly impacts on their loved ones (Broom and Kirby 2013). The many challenges posed by dying in turn reflect core discontents of modernity and contemporary social life. Giddens articulated this well in suggesting that a feature of modernity was that it purchas[ed] ontological security through institutions and routines that protect us from such things as criminality, madness … and *death*' (Giddens 1991; see also Willmott 2000, p. 649 for further discussion). With his words, we can begin to grasp how modernity can function to exclude questions that raise uncomfortable moral dilemmas, of which dying is a prime example (Willmott 2000: 649).

Dying is deeply unsettling to most. It poses uncomfortable questions around the purpose of our everyday lives, the importance of the 'self', as well as the legitimacy and even integrity of the structure of social organisation (Lee 2008; Willmott 2000). As Giddens and others since have outlined, dying is thus prone to being sequestered and, arguably, this process has been enhanced in the context of (late) modernity. Social life more broadly has become increasingly separated from existential concerns – including dilemmas around our mortality and the advent of death. Here, our cultural practices and institutions can be viewed as creative players in developing a 'protective' layer against the dread of the *meaning of life* particularly when put side-by-side with the *inevitability of death*.

As I have already alluded to, despite the (recent) historical tendency to sideline death and dying, there have been major shifts in recent years in terms of community awareness of, and the cultural visibility of, dying. Significant public debates and nuances in ways of understanding dying have developed (Walter 1999; Willmott 2000; Lee 2008). This has been facilitated by scholarly research revealing, among other things, the social circumstances of dying (for example, Clark 1993; Glaser and Strauss 1968; Kellehear 1990, 2008; Kubler-Ross 1969; Howarth 2007b; Lawton 2000; Seale 1998; Strauss 1970), and research exploring how experiences and perceptions of dying have shifted with the expansion and mainstreaming of palliative, hospice and end-of-life care (for example, James and Field 1992; Lawton 1998, 2000; McNamara 2001, 2004). Yet, despite this valuable scholarly contribution, and distinct improvements in the mainstreaming of the field, the dying process still conjures up stigma and despair, impacting at the very core of individual identities and our relationships with others. Moreover, how dying is increasingly being *done* in hospitals and hospices is challenging the traditional role of the family (for example, Broom and Kirby 2013; Kirby et al. 2014a) and the church (for example Bradshaw 1996; Brown 2009; Broom 2012a) in the dying process. This raises important questions about the expanding role of professions, institutions and the state in shaping experiences of death and dying (for example, Clark 2007; Hibbert et al. 2003; Stanley and Wise 2011). In turn, *how* and *where* people die is heavily shaped by ingrained forms of inequality and widening economic polarisation (for example, see Broom 2012a; House 2002). While Mark Twain considered death to be 'the great leveller', dying is certainly not, with class, gender and place, among other social dynamics, heavily influencing a person's 'ending', as well as their previous life chances up until death (Howarth 2007c; Broom 2012b). This raises broader questions around our agency, rights, forms of disadvantage, as well as the meaning and purpose of our everyday lives. In this way, I argue in this book that a critical sociological examination of dying must reflect as much on *how we live* as it does on *how we die*.

## Why a Social Perspective on Dying?

There is no one superior approach to analysing and interpreting the character and experience of dying within contemporary societies. Dying is investigated fruitfully in various fields like anthropology, ethics, philosophy, history, medicine and cultural studies among others. All of these fields have important contributions to make, which are vast and beyond the scope of this book. However, a sociological approach can uniquely get behind our cultural veneer in specific ways, for example, by highlighting the *shared experience* of dying, or by uncovering the *ideological underpinnings* of particular ways of dying. Moreover, a sociological approach reveals how dying involves unexpected twists and turns in the personal journey, the role of expertise, competing knowledges, varying moral framings and religious beliefs, on top of rapidly changing ways of organising death (Broom 2012a; Broom et al. 2013a, 2014b). To elucidate these social issues means treating dying as a meeting point between our social practices, institutions (for example, health care, family) and our individual biographies. Particularly, in the context of the interpretative traditions in sociology – which largely utilise qualitative and ethnographic methodologies – a sociological approach to dying can hold together *multiple truths* concurrently, treating professional, patient and family experiences as equally important, revealing and worthy of considered examination. As I hope to show in the following chapters, whether about doctors stubbornly holding onto hope, patients suffering in silence, nurses feeling unable to intervene in care, or families not acknowledging medical futility, a sociology of dying is about entertaining the whole messy picture to ask important questions like: *Why do such dynamics flourish?* and, *What are the implications for care practices and the various actors involved?*

One might argue that this is a well-trodden path with a significant amount of sociological and social science research and commentary exploring the area of death and dying already (some examples include Clark 1993; Glaser and Strauss 1968; Hockey 1990; Howarth 2007b; Kellehear 1984, 1990, 2008; Lawton 2000; Seale 1998). And yet, the interpersonal, community and organisational circumstances within which people are dying are rapidly changing, necessitating a reassessment of the social, economic and political contexts of dying across communities and cultures. As I explore in the following chapters, there are new and rising organisational and professional influences on the end of life, and these are continually remodelling (often imperceptibly at the individual level) the landscapes of dying in our communities and hospitals (see Broom and Cavenagh 2010; Broom et al. 2011, 2013a, 2013b, 2014a, 2014b). Moreover, there are evolving social expectations and reductive mindsets at play among professionals, and normative pressures on those who are nearing the end of their lives, with important consequences for the experience of dying and, indeed, the capacity for a 'good enough' death (see Broom 2009a; McClean

2005). Thus, a key contribution of this book is to highlight dying as *inter-subjective*, and that pathways towards, and choices at, the end of life involve multiple and negotiated subject positions, whether acknowledged by all actors or not (Broom et al. 2014b; MacArtney et al. 2014; Kirby et al. 2014a). In this way, stories of hope, acceptance, injustice and, importantly, experiences of suffering, peace and comfort at the end of life are necessarily co-written and co-starred in by a cast of patients, families, carers *and* professionals, and played out within the constraints and opportunities of the particular stage set for dying. Each player, as will become clear in the following chapters, participates in a complex social production of dying.

I should emphasise here that the following chapters utilise a critical sociological approach, but in a targeted fashion, exploring specific social dynamics and moments in care (often in formalised care settings). I do not seek to cover *all* spheres of dying or speak to experiences across all communities or cultural contexts. I focus almost exclusively on relations manifest in the context of illness and disease in Australia and at times the United Kingdom. So, for example, I do not seek to develop an understanding of the social dynamics of traumatic deaths (see Chapple and Ziebland 2015, for an excellent discussion), or other important sites of dying (like death in war, suicide, sudden deaths by road accident and so on). Instead I focus on dying from life-limiting illnesses, and caring for others in this particular situation. In gathering multi-stakeholder accounts of the dying process, I seek to explore what the implications are of dying in particular ways, in particular locations, surrounded by particular stakeholders, and supported by particular forms of expertise and governing rules. When taken together, the accounts that I have gathered and interpreted in this book tell us much about the evolving meanings of dying, and their implications for how we go about dying in modern Western societies.

## Situating Dying in Recent Historical and Social Context

Throughout the following chapters I focus on analysing experiences of dying – and caring for the dying – as relationally experienced, morally bound, and located in a cultural and historical context. It is perhaps useful then to provide a potted (albeit brief) historical account of dying in modern societies. There is considerable literature around the cultural reception of death and dying (for example, Beilin 1981; Becker 1973; Rousseau 2003; Zimmermann 2007), providing as it does a helpful scholarly and historical context to the chapters that follow. For instance, some scholars argued that death and dying created significant 'no go' areas in our social lives – coined *the death taboo*. The argument is that such dynamics have essentially come to frame the way we relate to death and dying. Denying our 'physical and symbolic mortality' became a core motivator of human conduct in modern societies (see Willmott 2000), including in the areas of sex and ageing. The death taboo thesis captured social anxieties around the inevitability of dying, connecting discontents around death with an emerging anomie and loss of meaning in modern societies (Lee 2008: 747). This dovetails nicely with Giddens's (1991) aforementioned argument around our deep needs to retain an ontological security in late modernity. As such, dying has become increasingly alarming in the context of modernity, especially given the (arguably) lack of meaningful and ritualistic structures surrounding it (Mellor and Shilling 1993; see also Lee 2008). The development of taboos around death and dying became an effective way of delineating between that which is prioritised in the West (self/life) and that which is not to be considered in everyday life (death/dying) (see Lee 2008: 650). The death taboo thus represents a crisis of meaning in modernity (Becker 1973; Lee 2008), instituting and protecting the boundary between living and dying (Giddens 1991: 156). I return to this debate around the death taboo, and questions around its contemporary relevance shortly. Before I do, it is useful to first consider a range of other economic, organisational and political influences that were important in framing understandings of, and approaches to, dying in the twentieth and now twenty-first centuries. The emergent anxieties of modernity around human mortality intertwined with, and were produced within, the context of various developments within the professional, institutional and political realms.

### *Improvements in Life Expectancy, Biomedical Development and Mastery of Disease*

The many biomedical and public health developments that functioned to dramatically extend the human life span heavily informed perceptions of dying in the twentieth century. Most babies born in 1900 did not live past age 50. Extraordinarily, in a little over a hundred years, life expectancy has been extended to over 80 years in a number of OECD countries (NIH 2011). Populations in early pre-industrial societies faced high risks of death with few people making it into what we would now consider 'old age'. The twentieth century's dramatic extension of life expectancy in the developed world, fuelled by biomedical responses to significant population killers (for example, smallpox, polio and measles), improvements in nutrition and public health and increasing social prosperity, contributed to a cultural mindset of mastery over disease (at least in theory) and an historic resiliency in the face of death (in practice). What emerged was an unprecedented shift toward *delaying death* (see also Kellehear 1984 on the 'death denying' society). It was increasingly assumed that each generation would, and could, live for longer and longer (Baltes and Smith 2003; Laslett 1991; Lubitz et al. 2003), with an emphasis on living and quality of life, rather than death and its qualities.

The surge in public confidence in scientific and biomedical development of the twentieth century coincided with, and contributed to a (partial and varied) secularisation of death and dying (Bradshaw 1996). While there are those who posit a recent 're-enchantment' of death and dying (for example, Lee 2008), it remains the case that there is much work to do in any re-appropriation of spirituality in the 'treatment' of death and dying metaphysically (cf. Bradshaw 1996). Essentially, dying from illness was gradually transformed over the course of the twentieth century into a *medical challenge* not just an *existential moment* (Emanuel and Emanuel 1998; Kubler-Ross 1969; Smith 2000; James and Field 1992; see also Cobb 2001). Increasingly medicalised, dying was drawn into various institutions and viewed as a site of medical expertise and professional skill (Clark 2002, 2007). While many individuals and groups within modern societies continued to espouse death-as-transition and dying-as-existential, scientific development and the medicalisation of everyday life encouraged an emphasis on the *mastery* of life and the body and a relation of *resistance* to death (Kellehear 1984; Zimmermann 2007).

Such socio-historical shifts were spurred on by political, medical and consumer developments that sought to 'conquer disease', and slow down the ageing process and bodily disintegration. This trajectory toward delaying ageing, mastering the body's unruly activities, and enhanced management of our 'lifestyles' to improve longevity, was furthered by the meteoric rise of biomedicine. Specific developments, including the discovery of antibiotics, blood transfusions, organ transplants, chemotherapeutic responses to cancer, and so forth, drove public faith in the potential for biomedical solutions to our bodily limits (Brenner 2002). The twentieth century was thus very much a century – until the later parts – centred on the seeming limitlessness of biomedicine in securing our existence, or at very least, significantly delaying death.

The dramatic rise in life expectancy in turn shifted the burden of disease. In doing so, it fundamentally altered the profile of death and dying across communities and societies (NIH 2011). Coined the 'epidemiological transition', this period was characterised by the waning of infectious and acute diseases in many economically richer societies and the emerging importance of chronic and degenerative diseases. People were less likely to be dying in their younger years of acute illnesses, but rather, were developing chronic illnesses over time and in older age (NIH 2011). This shift gave rise to palliative care, as many societies moved toward the medical management of pain and suffering in the context of longer periods of illness and, eventually, the management of the dying process.

### *Mastery of Disease, a Focus on Health, and Resistance to Death*

Responses to the rise of cancer with the 'epidemiological transition' provides a useful illustration of twentieth century responses to disease and life-limiting illness, with important flow-on effects for the broader reception of dying across societies (Chabner and Roberts 2005). America's 'war on cancer' of the Reagan era reflected a growing sense of humanity's capacity to eradicate disease – and the notion that achieving this was largely dependent on a combination of political will and economic means. The subsequent huge investment in biomedical therapeutic responses to cancer represented the peak of ambition to achieve its total eradication (Chabner and Roberts 2005). This political and medical ambition was met with some degree of despondency in the late twentieth century as early successes in curing certain cancers failed to result in its widespread eradication.

Despite the emerging realisation within the scientific community of the limits of the capacity of biomedical technologies to eradicate diseases such as cancer, public and political expectations remained high and a sense of the potential for persistent improvements in life-expectancy fed into a lack of focus on death, dying and bereavement. The human genome project represented yet another major development that promoted renewed hope that humanity would master disease, this time through understanding its genetics and developing targeted genetic solutions (cf. Petersen and Bunton 2002). These scientific trajectories provided a range of vital solutions to many health and illness problems, however, these activities were largely orientated toward *sustaining health*, rather than understanding and supporting death and dying.

These historical developments, in combination with the expansion of public healthcare in many OECD countries over the course of the twentieth century, meant an emerging civil society focus on the *right to health*, embedded in some degree of expectation of a 'good and long life', rather than the inevitability of dying. This was an important shift toward a wider discourse of *healthy citizenship* – a cultural shift that demanded new things of the modern state (that is, intervention and resource allocation) and of the individual (such as better lifestyle choices and self-management of health) that each would find difficult to fulfil (Petersen et al. 2010).

We can also see influences emerging from the political realm in terms of a lack of engagement with death and dying in modern societies. Discursive constructs, including 'healthy ageing', 'self-care', 'achieving wellbeing', and the '*third* age' rather than *old* age, all encourage longevity and resilience (Baltes and Smith 2003; see also Laslett 1991). Such sociocultural scripts are reflective of improving socioeconomic standards and an orientation toward wellness, and, in that sense, can be construed as largely positive. It is certainly true that enhanced opportunities for health, longevity and self-directed care, and their respective social scripts, can in certain circumstances be empowering, progressive and enabling. The problem emerges when the modern *healthy fixation* meets the limits of an individual's life course and the challenge of caring for the dying citizen with an unruly, disintegrating body (cf. Becker

1973; Beilin 1981; Rousseau 2003; Kellehear 1984; Zimmerman 2007). This is where cultural ideas about the value of resilience, longevity and wellbeing may not necessarily produce productive outcomes. Culturally, life is simply more palatable than death for most of us, and getting more of it is a core modern desire, placing dying in a challenging and interpersonal cultural space.

There are also underlying and emerging economic dimensions to dying. Whether dying at home or in an institution, it can be expensive for the individual and for the modern state whether paid for through public healthcare provision or indirectly through state subsidised private insurers (Elsayem et al. 2004; Emanuel and Emanuel 1994; Morrison et al. 2008; Smith et al. 2003). With increasing numbers of people dying within institutions rather than in the home (see also Exley and Allen 2007), and enhanced privatisation of healthcare services, there is significant potential for dying to be increasingly economically mediated, with the level of care provided at home or in an institution partially determined by the level of healthcare cover, or for heightened rationing of resources to support dying within public health systems. In the Australian context, for example, people with private insurance and good economic resources have access to advanced in-patient palliative care services that those with fewer resources would not. Dying should thus be viewed as situated within the broader shift toward neoliberalism and a retraction of the state in times of economic austerity. Delaying death thus delays the associated costs of dying, offering an additional (economic) mediating factor at the end of life.

Given the economic burden of the dying process and the benefits of delaying death, it is a prerogative of the modern state to encourage resilient citizens who work hard and live long and healthy lives, thus lowering the overall economic burden on the state (see CDC 2005 for reduced productivity from smoking). Despite ambiguities around how much such strategies actually save health service providers economically (for example, Lubitz et al. 2003), the modern state relies heavily on the promotion of 'longer', 'healthier' and 'productive' lives. Such structural conditions promoting health, self-sufficiency and longevity, can have the effect of shifting the focus away from dying and caring for the dying amongst families and communities.

According to Lee (2008), the late twentieth and early twenty-first centuries have witnessed significant allaying of taboo around death and dying, citing an 'over-generalisation of a social fear around death and the failure to address the shifting context of death discourse' (Lee 2008, p. 748; see also Walter 1999; Willmott 2000). In many respects I concur with this assessment, particularly the argument that the notions of a 'death taboo' can create an overly linear social relation around death and dying, lacking nuance across individuals, communities and cultures. Certainly, there is little doubt that the growth of hospice and palliative care have contributed greatly to enhancing public understandings, and the broader cultural visibility, of dying. Moreover, there are new spiritualities and ways of understanding death and dying which disrupt the medicalisation of dying thesis. Yet, I would argue that new social movements and professional developments in the field have themselves created new and, at times, problematic structures for dying as well as reinforcing, to some extent, the sidelining of dying in modern society (see Chapters 3 and 4 for in-depth discussion of this). As Lee argues, concepts of death taboo and death denial can be overstated, and that there are various reconfigurations of death and dying in modernity that are not merely about practices of denial, sequestering and alienation (Lee 2008: 748). For Lee there has been revolt against the trappings of modernity, including the re-enchantment of dying through new forms of pluralism and emerging spiritualities (Lee 2008: 756). Lee's work emphasises the importance of not reifying cultural taboos around death and dying and maintaining sensitivity to new and emerging ritual practices which move beyond dread and the practice of sequestering. This is certainly relevant to the work presented in the following chapters.

While it may be true that death and dying are no longer strictly taboo, and that dying has gained much more visibility over the course of the twentieth and now twenty-first centuries, there remains a need to place more emphasis on mainstreaming and normalising the end of life. The problem, as I will argue in the following chapters, is that while we are provided a plenitude of advice and support for healthy living in modern societies, there is a paucity of awareness and understanding of dying and the various possibilities surrounding the dying process (Emanuel and Emanuel 1998; Smith 2000; Steinhauser et al. 2000). Even in the context of serious life-limiting illness, care tends to be orientated around *living with* illness and disability, and the value of survivorship, rather than the meanings and normalcy of dying. Enter palliative, hospice and end-of-life care providers and practitioners – fields of healthcare which are critical foci of this book. These relatively new sites of organisational support and expertise are charged with preparing many of us for and assisting us in the dying process. This, as will already be clear, is no easy task (see also Hibbert et al. 2003), and some reflection on the historical, political and social influences on the development of these fields is useful.

While I have only provided a short, and selective, historical background, the purpose has been to illustrate how the economic, political and social can dovetail to encourage particular sensibilities around death and dying – some of which are related to entirely natural human characteristics toward embracing life (Rousseau 2003; Seale 1998; Zimmermann 2007). The institutional and organisational dynamics of dying are worthy of further consideration, including how the twentieth century witnessed a surge in interest in and support for formalised palliative and end-of-life care.

### *The Rise and Significance of Palliative Care: The Institutions and Professions of Dying*

The aforementioned cultural and historical shifts are intimately intertwined with major shifts in caring for the dying. The rise of specialist palliative care[1] represented a radical shift in how dying was done internationally (Clark 2002, 2007). In pre-modern contexts, dying largely occurred within the home, and care was provided by family and/or non-kin caregivers. Moreover, dying was intimately enmeshed with forms of religiosity, with religious organisations instilling meaning around the purpose of death and dying. Dying in religious terms was/is a rite of passage and a transition to an existential realm. While the path may have been one involving significant suffering, the end result is conceived as one of peace or rest (depending on the particular life lived). In the context of surging public support for science, and the rise of medicalisation, dying as the exclusive domain of the church, or other religious organisations, did not match the evolving cultural environment of the twentieth and twenty-first centuries. For example, in the current Australian context on which I often focus in this book, over 22 per cent of the population report 'no religion' (2011 Census data) and projections based on present trends indication that 'no religion' will be the most popular response by the next census. While this may be very different from the mid-twentieth century within which palliative and hospice care was emerging or becoming formalised (Clark 2002, 2007), a broad (albeit contested) shift toward the secularisation of societies has been indicated for quite some time (Brown 2009; Turner 2011; see also Bradshaw 1996). This has

1 *Specialist palliative care* refers to services provided by an interdisciplinary team of specialist palliative care professionals whose substantive work is with patients who have an eventually fatal condition (PCA 2010). Palliative care, as defined by the World Health Organization, is an approach that improves the quality of life of patients and their families facing the problems associated with life threatening illness, through the prevention and relief of suffering by means of early identification, impeccable assessment, and treatment of pain and other problems – physical, psychosocial, and spiritual (WHO 2004; see also Mitchell 2011). Palliative care is delivered in varying ways and by a range of healthcare professions, including those working in general practice settings, hospitals and hospices (Mitchell 2011). In Australia, in larger metropolitan hubs, specialist palliative care units exist to provide comprehensive specialised in-patient and community-based palliative care. The majority of patients are initially referred to such units by medical specialists rather than GPs. Once referred, GPs may continue to provide support within a shared care model. Palliative care may also be provided pre-referral to a specialist unit, particularly in contexts where a patient has an established relationship with their medical specialist and limited palliative care needs. Cancer patients constitute around 80 per cent of the palliative care patient population in Australia (Mitchell 2011).

been reflected in turn in dying being increasingly viewed as a site of medical and health expertise that requires clinical and institutional management, rather than largely as an individual's *existential struggle* to be managed by family, community and religious organisations (see also Hibbert et al. 2003). Dying has become significantly diversified in terms of public versus private 'management' (that is, home versus institution), and in terms of the range of stakeholders (for example, religious, spiritual, medical, supportive care focused) potentially involved in the process (Bradshaw 1996). Moreover, the forms of spiritual and religious input provided at the end of life are shifting, diversifying and are even now embedded in the priorities and histories of the specific organisations providing formalised care. This provides both *plural/liberative* and *disruptive/normative* potential. As Lee (2008: 748) states, 'in an age of increasing secularisation where God is seen to have departed ... the concept of death becomes even more critical as it can no longer be presumed that death is simply the preserve of divinity'.

The rise of specialist palliative care[2] is a very recent phenomenon and represents an important new site for sociological inquiry. For example, it was not until 1998 that palliative medicine became a formal medical specialty in Australia with advanced trainee opportunities (Clark 2002, 2007). While nursing and general practice had longstanding interests and involvement in palliative and end-of-life care, the formalisation of a unique and new medical specialty in its own right differentiated it from other fields of medicine, and placed more value on end-of-life training, initiating a shift in healthcare resources, increased capacity to deliver, and greater recognition of, end-of-life care. Prior to this, palliative care was often done in an ad hoc fashion, delivered in non-systematic ways by (non-specialised) treating physicians, general practitioners (GPs) in the community and nurses (for example, Field 1989). The rise of palliative care, and the greater penetration of palliative care into the hospital sector, fundamentally shifted the management and experience of dying (Hart, Sainsbury and Short 1998; Hibbert et al. 2003).

While dying was becoming increasingly located and managed as an illness or disease experience rather than an existential moment, shifts towards dying as a 'medical event' have been complicated by the fact that the roots of much hospice care (at least in the Australian and British contexts) lie firmly in Anglo-Christian values regarding the existential meanings of dying (for example, Broom 2012a). These values may include those of gift, sacrifice, rites of passage and acceptance, among others (for example, Froggatt 1997). What this has meant, certainly in

2 There is some variability in what these terms mean across national contexts. In Australia 'hospice' refers to end-of-life care in an in-patient unit. In the US 'hospice' refers to a programme where patients are cared for at home. In the UK a 'hospice' can be a specific site including in-patients and out-patients and the broader multifaceted care.

the Australian context, is that while the rise of palliative care in the mid to late twentieth century shifted the emphasis toward dying as a *medical moment* (Hibbert et al. 2003), the hospice movement continued to espouse (albeit often implicitly) a range of Anglo-Christian scripts around dying and utilise these within the delivery of care (cf. Bradshaw 1996; see also Broom 2012a). While there are sites of diversity, and constant diversification within palliative and hospice care, there remain persistent ideological influences which are worthy of consideration. As scholars have previously pointed out, these included values around acceptance and stoicism in the end of life, with *dying well* illustrative of personal strength and character (for example, Hart, Sainsbury and Short 1998; McNamara 2004). This has meant an interesting and at times problematic mix, as I examine in Chapter 4, of ongoing religious *and* professional influences on experiences of dying in palliative and end-of-life settings (Broom 2012a; Broom and Cavenagh 2010, 2011; Hart, Sainsbury and Short 1998; Nissim et al. 2009).

Regardless of the complexities presented by the medicalisation of dying of the mid to late twentieth century (explored in subsequent chapters), the gradual rise of specialist palliative and hospice care resulted in significantly more options being made available to people at the end of life (Clark 2002, 2007). However, this also created a concern amongst social scientists around what an institutional death would look like versus dying at home or in other community settings (Bradshaw 1996; Stanley and Wise 2011). Significant questions quickly emerged around the capacity of biomedicine to adequately deal with dying *outside* of the home (Illick 1976; James and Field 1992) and the threat of biomedical institutions providing restrictive and alienating forms of care at the end of life (Howarth 2007). The notion of the *social death* captured some aspects of this dynamic, including processes of institutionalisation that result in the removal of a person from social life, thus resulting in a pre-death of sorts (see Howarth 2007b for further discussion).

Further questions were raised as palliative and hospice care increased in prominence, including what new forms of dying were being *imposed* on patients and their families (James and Field 1992; Hart, Sainsbury and Short 1998; Mellor and Shilling 1990; Lawton 1998, 2000; Walter 1999). Sociologists were growing increasingly concerned that the emerging field of 'palliative medicine' might risk the sequestering of the dying process, further stigmatising and separating it from everyday life (Stanley and Wise 2011; see also Broom and Cavenagh 2011). The medicalisation of dying – via hospice and specialist palliative care – from this angle had potential to reinforce the cultural dispositions toward death denial, separating those who are dying from the community and their families, and further concealing this important point in the life course (see also Mellor and Shilling 1993). Furthermore, there was a significant concern that the medicalisation of dying would remove the existential and mystical from the dying process – that we were on a path toward the widespread routinisation of dying (Bradshaw 1996; James and Field 1992). What emerged was a tension between the necessary formalisation and systematisation of palliative and end-of-life care (to augment life-prolonging options), and the desire to recognise and 'treat' dying as a social, cultural and spiritual occasion, not just a medical problem (Broom and Cavenagh 2011; Seale 1998). These tensions are quite clearly evident in the following chapters through the accounts of those who are dying.

### *The Contemporary Context: Palliation, Professions and Problematising the Medical Focus on Life-Prolongment*

While in many respects, processes of professionalisation and mainstreaming within the palliative and hospice care movement have improved care of the dying, as will be illustrated in the following chapters, they have also raised important questions regarding the relationship between different medical and allied health professions and sites of expertise. The significant expansion of specialist palliative care in the hospital sector and into the community in Australia (and in other contexts) has introduced new logics, practices and priorities into health service delivery. Those heavily involved in specialist palliative care are strongly emphasising early transitions and referrals to palliative care, as well as the normalisation and de-stigmatisation of the dying process more broadly. A recent ground-breaking study by Temel et al. (2010) showed that much earlier transitions to palliative care improved quantity of life (survival) and quality of life, resulting in sustained critique of the well-documented tendencies of doctors significantly delaying referrals to palliative care, evident across the hospital sector (Broom et al. 2013a, 2014b). While this particular study was focusing on lung cancer, it challenged the often implicit medical practice of resisting medical futility and not facilitating timely transitions to palliative care – a process regularly ascribed to a resistance to 'giving up' from patients and families. As will be shown in Chapter 2, doctors play critical roles in such dynamics in the pursuit of life-prolongment.

Despite such evidence around the importance to timely transitions, the roll-out and expansion of specialist palliative care services has continued to jar with the persistent life-prolonging foci of many doctors working in the non-palliative trained medical specialties (Broom et al. 2013a, 2014a, 2014b) and created new problematic dynamics across the health sector. My ongoing research in collaboration with other colleagues has shown that specialist palliative and supportive care nurses in hospital contexts are increasingly challenging others within nursing (and in medicine) to invest more time and energy in palliative and end-of-life issues (e.g. Broom et al. 2014a; Kirby et al. 2014b), yet power relations and professional dynamics are limiting their capacity to influence practices (see Chapter 6, 'Nursing the Dying'). Specialist palliative care doctors are taking similar steps, and are being confronted by complex inter-professional relations across palliative versus life-prolonging sectors of medicine (see Chapter 2, 'Time to Die').

The last two decades have thus witnessed a dramatic series of changes in the dying professions and care of the dying, with enhanced professional legitimacy in palliative medicine, cultural visibility of caring for the dying, clearer purpose and priorities within these communities of practice, but has also presented significant challenges in relation to resonance within other sectors of medicine and health care priorities more broadly. Yet, while the mainstreaming of palliative and end-of-life care has in some respects 'outed' dying as not the horror it once was considered, raising its profile within communities, dying and the end of life still receive relatively little attention in the public sphere. Forms of advocacy and support seen in other illness contexts (for example, cancer survivorship or disability support) are certainly not evident in palliative and end-of-life care. Dying does not provide the 'good news stories' we are so often presented with in other contexts. The question of why *resistance to death* continues is complex and multi-faceted, and it remains the case, as I explore in the following chapters, that when faced with death, much of the horror and fear is simply not evident. It becomes an important task for social scientists to disentangle social and cultural discontents and the actual character of individual experiences (and their intersections). Palliative care reveals as much about life, and our social mores, concerns and fears, as it does about how we view 'death' as the medical end point. As I shall illustrate in the following chapters, in the last few weeks of life, for many people the dying process may engender gift, peace and contentment (see Chapter 3, 'Places for Dying'). This too is an authentic and common experience of dying (see MacArtney et al. 2014), and provides a balance to what is often conceived of as a fraught process characterised by loss and grief.

Resistance to death continues to underpin, or is implicit in, much interaction within clinical and community settings. Some doctors, as we see in Chapter 2 ('Time to Die'), attempting to master disease and delay the body's inevitable disintegration, can contribute to a culture of death denial or resistance to the shift to end-of-life care (see also Campbell et al. 2010; The et al. 2000). Families and informal carers are also participants in the broader construction of resilience and the omnipotence of human persistence, at times co-producing a morality of survival and resistance to death (see Chapters 4 and 5). More recently, some complementary and alternative medicine (CAM) practitioners and 'cancer gurus' have been complicit in the drive for survival and longevity, even in the context of advanced, incurable disease (see Chapter 7, 'Dying, Healing and Survivorship'), offering new therapeutic potential but also new previously unexplored normativities in end-of-life contexts. All stakeholders, I argue in this book, are important 'players' in the way dying is done and in perpetuating the social scripts that circulate around those facing the end of life. Families and friends – and their ideas about the 'good fight' and the importance of 'staying around' – further feed the desire for life and resistance to death (Kirby et al. 2014a, MacArtney et al. 2014; see also Kellehear 2008). While resilience, struggle and fight can be highly agentive practices for many people, when the underlying relation is one of the abhorrence of death, dying can produce extraordinarily difficult emotions and tense social relations; multi-stakeholder resistance to *death* – particularly if unrecognised and merely underlying social relations – can significantly problematise the dying process.

Throughout this book I will unpack what this means and looks like in the contemporary context, including the role of hope, normativity and the agentive aspects of deaths allowed and deaths denied. As I outline in the following chapters, dying can be an important site of control, oppression, transcendence and resistance; it plays out the classic sociological dilemmas of power, agency and submission. It is prone to inequality whereby those with greater opportunities, resources and literacy may question and resist normative frameworks to a greater extent. Rather than being a great leveller, dying reflects persistent social relations of injustice and marginality (see also Broom and Cavenagh 2010; Broom, Good et al. 2013c; Seymour et al. 2007); the practice of dying is reflective of one's capacity to engage with, draw on, and resist available ideas and resources.

## The Fieldwork

This book relies on periods of fieldwork in Australia (late 2000s to present) and in the United Kingdom (mid-2000s). The period of research in Britain involved the collection of qualitative data from the National Health Service (NHS) cancer patients (see Chapter 7, 'Dying, Healing and Survivorship'). I returned to Australia in the late 2000s and completed a series of qualitative studies focused on the experiences of advanced cancer patients in the community, as well as patients with a range of illnesses in the last four weeks of life receiving in-patient hospice care. This later period of data collection was the most important for driving my own interest in the area of end-of-life care and features strongly within the following chapters: Chapter 3, 'A Place for Dying', Chapter 4, 'The Moralities and Politics of Dying', Chapter 8, 'Gender and the Moralities of Dying' and Chapter 9, 'The Dying Body'. In particular, a group of participants residing in a New South Wales (Australia) hospice gave me the most significant insight into the last few weeks of life, as they recounted inspirational, challenging and at times frightening stories of living and dying in the hospice. Their stories prompted me to engage in further periods of fieldwork with other patients, families and health professionals in Queensland (Australia), some of which are still underway at the time of writing this book. The period of research with patients in New South Wales also prompted me to move my research focus to include clinical perspectives and health professionals' accounts of their own emotions at the point of futility and at the end of life. Data collection for fieldwork with health professionals took place from 2012 until 2014 and features in Chapters 2 ('Time to Die') and 6 ('Nursing the Dying').

## A Note on Researching Dying

These periods of fieldwork across Australia and Britain involved significant work to develop a sensitive research strategy suitable for vulnerable populations. The research process was both rewarding and challenging both for me and the participants. The fieldwork brought with it a whole series of questions around the relationship of the researcher to the researched; what could be tolerated in terms of interview questions, what could be justified in terms of fieldwork, and what lay within the parameters of each research project and period of fieldwork (Johnson and Clarke 2003). People regularly ask me, 'Why do you research dying, doesn't it depress you?'. That dying and the end of life would be considered in such negative terms reflects much about the cultural reception and perception of dying, and says little about the actual process of dying itself. As shown in the following chapters, dying can be extraordinarily difficult but it can also be meaningful, and ultimately, timely, with positive and empowering elements. As a researcher I was exposed to the spectrum of emotions – elation, peace, hopelessness, anger and despair. I certainly felt the injustice, untimeliness and suffering of some of my participants' situations. Researching dying in turn presents you with your own existential questions which are not easily resolved. But any adverse effects are countered by the fact that your own fears illustrate that it is an important social problem and, moreover, that you are able to connect with the (often acute) experience of nearing the end of life.

Dying is a universal experience that eventually impacts on every family and every person. Over the course of writing this book I was faced with a terminal illness and subsequent death in my own family. This created issues for me in terms of balancing my academic interest in dying and a parallel process in my personal life. That experience continues to shape my academic work and how I reflect on it. The themes emergent in the following chapters – of gross injustice, horror, fear, resilience and acceptance – resonated biographically for me during this period of study. While immensely difficult at times, I found this parallel experience facilitated greater connection with the participants' stories and certainly resulted in me being more attuned than I otherwise would be to their dilemmas, difficulties, sites of suffering and individual journeys toward the end of life. The following chapters are based on the results of studies largely involving in-depth interviews. Given that the participants (other than the professionals and carers) were within months, if not weeks, of death, I took extreme care to ensure that 'collecting data' was always secondary to participant wellbeing, dignity and comfort (Liamputtong 2006). It was heartening that the participants almost unanimously fed back to me and to other staff that their participation was not overly burdensome, was sometimes therapeutic, and even enjoyable at times.

## Outline of the Chapters

Chapter 2, *Time to Die? Breaking the News of Futility and the End of Life*, focuses on senior specialist doctors' accounts of discussing futility and topicalising dying with their patients. In particular I examine the dilemmas faced by doctors in hospital contexts in 'bringing up' palliative care and the dying process more broadly. I focus on the logics underpinning dialogue, how they experience acknowledging futility, and how they go about talking about dying. I utilise their accounts to reveal the emotional and inter-subjective influences on recognising futility and initiating palliative care, positioning doctors as complicit in the co-production of hope and resistance to 'letting go'. In *Time to Die?* I posit that doctors are an under-examined site of the production of hope *and* resistance to dying, and that a focus on their emotional and subjective influences is urgently needed.

Chapter 3, *A Place for Dying*, engages with questions around the contemporary location of dying, focusing on the institutional inflection of the dying process, including personal and interpersonal dilemmas around the hospice context. This chapter, drawing on qualitative research with people in the last few weeks of life, considers the relative experiential benefits of dying in a hospice. This chapter considers both the benefits and limitations of institutionalised dying, providing an explication of how place is crucial to the experience and character of dying. I argue in *A Place for Dying* that the hospice allows certain possibilities (that is, hope, play and a space for living) but also presents unique challenges to the individual (that is, liminal spheres and pressure to be 'accomplished' in death). Moreover, the hospice as an institution provides significant insight into social and cultural discontents around death, dying and human mortality.

Chapter 4, *The Moralities and Politics of Dying in a Hospice*, focuses in on the role of institutional moralities in shaping the dying process, including the ethical and normative frameworks people can be exposed to. I focus on the dynamics of 'assisted dying' and 'religiosity' within the hospice environment and how they articulate important aspects of the institutional governance of dying. I utilise ideas about the moral economy of caring and dying to capture the governance of 'timely' and 'good' deaths. In doing this I argue that such 'social contracts' at the end of life concurrently allow certain possibilities and limit human agency, and that the modern hospice represents the bureaucratisation of the 'timely death' buttressed by a religiously framed transitional mode of 'exit' from this world. The threat, I posit, is that some hospices may function to marginalise alternative ways of dying and provide a series of constraints on ways of dying in an institutional context.

Chapter 5, *Families and Dying*, shifts the focus toward relations of informal care and the powerful role of the family and non-kin caregivers in the overall cultural production of dying. With significant shifts in individual roles within families and family structures over the twentieth century, dying is increasingly shaped by important cultural transitions including weakening family ties (i.e. ontological insecurity) and moves toward individualisation. I focus on moving beyond the family as merely a 'stakeholder in care', to the family as complicit in the production of dying, and implicitly or explicitly encouraging certain trajectories. I argue here that dying can only be understood from within a framework that incorporates the dynamics of informal care and tensions between individual desires and family values and needs.

In Chapter 6, *Nursing the Dying*, I focus on the role of nursing in the transition to palliative and end-of-life care. I argue that nurses are precariously positioned as *intimate mediators* in the context of dying, required to gain necessary interpersonal intimacy with their patients whilst doing 'technical nursing' and maintaining 'professional distance'. I illustrate how nurses are involved in ensuring a sentimental order within the hospital whereby emotions around futility and dying are kept at manageable levels for various stakeholders including doctors, patients and families. While the interviews illustrate that nursing capital lies within the particular intimate relations they maintain with patients and families, they also considered themselves entrapped within a medical–nursing hierarchy. This means that despite nurses having an awareness of futility and the urgent need for palliative care (and awareness of dying), this was resisted by doctors, and nursing knowledge thereby sidelined. I argue that formalising and enhancing the role of nurses will inevitably improve transitions to the end of life and experiences of dying.

In Chapter 7, *Dying, Healing and Survivorship*, I engage with contestations around dying and terminality, focusing on the enactment of resistance to a 'terminal' diagnosis and the emerging role of CAM and 'cancer gurus' therein. In particular I examine the rise of *survivorship* in the context of advanced terminal cancer, and how the proliferation of CAM and modern 'cancer gurus' has contributed to a reframing of the experience of 'being terminal'. While I outline the importance of agency invoking practices of self-care and self-healing, I also find within such processes a problematic normativity espousing virtue, control and individual responsibility. I argue that 'alternative' survivorship is a contemporary inflection point in dying, presenting emancipatory *and* normative potential for those embarking on a journey post diagnosis of 'advanced, terminal cancer'. Such 'survivorship' discourses, moralities of resilience, and practices of resistance have significant flow-on effects for health professionals and families who are seeking to provide formal and informal care as the end of life nears.

Chapter 8, *Gender and the Moralities of Dying*, focuses on some intersections of gender identities and the dying process. Continuing the previous chapters' themes around moralities and the relationality of dying, here I embark on an explication of how gendered dynamics can strongly mediate expectations, obligations and responsibilities at the end of life. These impact on those who are dying and those who care for them. While there is a plenitude of biographical variables influencing the experience of dying (for example, class and ethnicity), I view gender as a particularly under-researched area of death and dying, and thus worthy of significant focus. There has been a general tendency within the social sciences to interpret end-of-life experiences as largely undifferentiated in their bodily and emotional impact, and thus, I argue that a more nuanced conception of dying is necessary; exploring the role of masculinities is a starting point. I outline the importance of disentangling the intersectionality of moral practice and gender identities, arguing that gendered interpersonal dynamics are complicit in the production of virtuous 'good deaths'.

In Chapter 9, *The Dying Body*, I explore the embodied experience of dying, with a focus on the lived experience of managing the disintegrating body at the end of life. I explore cultural sensibilities around the body and relations of disgust, and how such ideas may inflect experiences of dying. More than merely a matter of suffering, pain or discomfort, our dying bodies are socially and relationally unsettling, with medical practices utilised to cope with, and ameliorate, this confronting process of bodily disintegration. Mapping lived experiences of lack of bodily control, and individual accounts of bodily disintegration, I illustrate how what the body does at the end of life is socially meaningful, not merely a physiological reality. The dying body raises a wide range of discontents around the body and the borders of the body, heavily inflecting formal and informal care of the dying, and reflect on our modern sensibilities around sanitisation and repulsion with waste. I consider how we treat and experience disordered bodies at the end of life, practices of resistance to the final acts of the body, and the dynamics of receiving care in the context of bodily disintegration. I suggest that further attention should be paid to embodied relations at the end of life, and the potential for both suffering and comfort.

In Chapter 10 I outline a targeted future research agenda for the sociological study of dying, including reflecting on the limits of the analyses presented in the book and areas for expansion. I note areas of significant neglect, particularly death and dying in the developing world, and the importance of expanding the social study of the end of life across borders and socioeconomic strata. Dying has been a persistently neglected area of care and this book provides a series of targeted analyses which require international comparative work to fully comprehend the complexities and cultural nuances of our lives and deaths.

# Chapter 2
# Time to Die? Breaking the News of Futility and the End of Life

## Introduction

I begin the empirical chapters of this book with a focus on doctors and their experiences of the rather challenging point in clinical care when questions around futility begin to emerge and the transition to the end of life becomes increasingly difficult to 'put off', so to speak. Part of the reason I begin with this particular clinical moment is that it is significantly under-examined and yet critical to initiating the transition to end of life and the dying process. It is also what often stands in the way of a timely and effective transition to palliative and/or end-of-life care. Within the existing literature it has generally been the *initial* diagnosis with cancer (or some other life-limited illness) that has been treated as the pivotal clinical moment for the patient, families and professionals. Yet, I argue that it is often the *point of medical futility* and an emerging awareness of the lack of meaningful life-prolonging therapeutic options that poses the greatest challenge for patients and their doctors (Arnold and Egan 2004; Burt 2002; Campbell et al. 2010; Clayton et al. 2005; Friedrichsen and Strang 2003; Hanratty et al. 2012; Lofmark, Nilstun and Bolmsjo 2005).

This is the clinical moment – or series of moments – where the *idea of dying* moves to centre stage, heavily inflecting interactions and introducing a multitude of emotional and existential dilemmas (Zimmermann 2007). This moment has rarely been explored within the sociological literature; rather, social scientists – as with the health and medical literature – have firmly placed the emphasis on being told 'your illness is terminal' rather than being told 'you're dying' (The et al. 2000; VandeKieft 2001; Wittenberg-Lyles et al. 2008).

Given the paucity of critical analysis on the dynamics of topicalising and communicating futility, I begin this book with an examination of a group of Australian doctors' perspectives on managing the emerging realisation of medical futility and, in turn, their experiences of topicalising dying with patients and their families. In particular, I focus on how some doctors manage this potentially fraught interpersonal dynamic, their emotions and the subsequent complex conversations about the end of life. In some cases this includes explication of their own resistance to initiating discussions about palliative or end-of-life care and the dying process more broadly. I draw on their stories of clinical interactions to illustrate that *interpersonal discontents* and *emotional subjectivities* play a central role in the recognition of dying and thus pathways to the end of life (for example, Arnold and Egan 2004; Friedrichsen and Strang 2003; Morita et al. 2004; Quill, Arnold and Back 2009). Yet, so often these relational processes are sidelined in the scholarly literature. My analysis of doctors' accounts in this chapter is augmented in subsequent chapters where I focus on patient accounts of the transition to, and experiences of, palliative and end-of-life care (see Chapters 3 and 4). Consistent with the broader analysis developed in this book, I argue in this chapter that recognition of dying is highly relational and intersubjective, and that clinical encounters (and pathways to the end of life) are strongly shaped by socio-cultural ideas around injustice, hope and a broader resistance to mortality.

## Background

### *The Troubles of Futility and Managing Transitions to the End of Life*

Acknowledging that patients are dying and then initiating palliative care can be challenging for doctors (Brickner et al. 2004; Campbell et al. 2010; Friedman, Harwood and Shields 2002; Johnson et al. 2008). While the issues individual doctors face can vary substantially (Hardy et al. 2008; Heedman and Starkhammar 2002; see also Ahmed et al. 2004), it is clear that these clinical moments are prone to interpersonal and emotional difficulties both for doctors and for their patients (Salander 2002; Thorne et al. 2006; The et al. 2000; Smith et al. 2010). Senior doctors, or medical specialists in the Australian context, have ultimate responsibility for negotiating and communicating futility and the need for end-of-life care (Christakis 1999). The key challenges they face include the emotional aspects of communicating 'bad news', the uncertainty around futility and in deciding the point of transition from life-prolonging to life-enhancing care, and the desire to provide hope within the context of terminality (Brown et al. 2009; Ronaldson and Devery 2001; Smith et al. 2010, Smith et al. 2012). Previous work provides some indication that conversations about the shift to palliative and/or end-of-life care are influenced by personality and relationship factors (Hagerty et al. 2005; Maynard 1996; Ptacek and Eberhardt 1996; Salander 2002; The et al. 2000; Thorne et al. 2006; Walshe et al. 2008). Furthermore, clinical decision making around hope versus futility can vary between individual clinicians (Broom and Adams 2010). Hitherto we have only limited understanding of the inter-subjective and emotional issues that may shape the process and experience of discussions around futility and dying. How do emotions, subjectivities and biomedical culture mediate awareness, recognition and eventually the experience of dying?

## *Dying and Emotions*

The subjectivities and emotionality of medical work have been of interest in the sociology of health and illness for quite some time (for example, Fox 1959; Fox and Lief 1963; Graham 2006; James 1989; Lupton 1997; Nettleton, Burrows and Watt 2008; Wallace and Lemaire 2007). Early research produced a range of important concepts that speak to the contemporary issues faced in palliative care contexts. Fox and Lief's (1963) notion of *detached concern* captured the precarious balance of empathy and detachment in medical training and medical work, and the potential for over-detachment and mechanistic treatment of patients. Freidson's (1988) research on the *clinical mentality* also contributed significantly to our understanding of clinical work within the context of emotion and subjectivity, including how the clinical mentality (that is, a focus on clinical experience, belief, 'making a difference', faith, 'doing good' and so on) can promote an activist orientation in treating patients (Freidson 1988). This represented an epistemological individualism; a systematic bias operating concurrently with rationality. The notion of *sentimental work* (Strauss et al. 1982) sought to capture the dialectic between the emergent techno-scientific workplace and human emotion, providing a basis for understanding the management of emotion/s in response to instrumental work within the hospital. Sentimental work, it was argued, personalises medicine in a highly depersonalised institutional environment, situating medical practice within implicit and explicit understandings of the interpersonal and the contextual (Strauss et al. 1982: 254). This resonates with the sociology of emotions more broadly, including work of Hochschild (1983), which revealed the ways in which emotions are *both* performed (as part of work) and managed or absorbed (as part of professional coping mechanisms). In sum, the management of emotions has been viewed for some time as a vital but often under-recognised feature of medical practice, concurrently acting as a potential resource, an impediment and a challenge, and most importantly, from a sociological standpoint, as framing the delivery of care.

While emotions in medicine remain an important theme within the contemporary sociological literature (for example, Graham 2006; Nettleton, Burrows and Watt 2008; Wallace and Lemaire 2007), as Nettleton, Burrows and Watt (2008: 20) point out, 'there is a relative "silence" about feelings when doctors talk to researchers, or indeed when researchers talk to doctors'. This dynamic, they argue, is associated with the sense within medicine, and imbued in the psyche of many doctors, that feelings are risky in that they threaten the abstract system of medicine (Nettleton, Burrows and Watt 2008). Whether or not this is the case, there still remains a paucity of sociological research exploring accounts of emotion and inter-subjectivity from the perspectives of doctors. This is an important area of enquiry in end-of-life contexts given the potentially heightened human emotions and subjective influences.

## *The End of Life and the Role of Emotion*

Research across academic disciplines provides some insight into the ways in which *discussions about futility and dying* in particular are embedded in emotional and inter-subjective challenges (for example, Arnold and Egan 2004; Friedrichsen and Strang 2003; Morita et al. 2004; Quill, Arnold and Back 2009). The et al.'s (2000) study of small cell lung cancer patients, for example, illustrates how some doctors embark on *medical activism* to help them and their patients divide the illness trajectory into much smaller, less emotionally charged, and more optimistic end points (The et al. 2000). This speaks to the potential co-production of optimism stemming from inclinations towards collusion that are embedded in emotionality and relationality in medical contexts (Zimmermann 2007; see also Smith et al. 2012). Given the potential for emotion and sentimentality, how then is the need for palliative care and the dying process topicalised and experienced by doctors? Facilitating this shift toward the end of life care is challenging (see Brickner et al. 2004; Friedman, Harwood and Shields 2002; Hibbert et al. 2003; Lofmark, Nilstun and Bolmsjo 2005; Quill, Arnold and Back 2009). Negotiations are highly individualised as well as multifactorial, including patient preparedness, conceptions of risk and benefit, family desire, and so on (Bestall et al. 2004). The 'point of futility' is a notoriously grey area, precariously positioned between clinical judgement and historical predictors of survival (Friedman, Harwood and Shields 2002; Heedman and Starkhammar 2002). Compounding these challenges, the shift to palliation or end-of-life care presents doctors with dilemmas around the patient's right to all available treatment, the importance of maintaining hope, and the ethics of withdrawing 'technically' life-prolonging options (Melvin and Oldham 2009; Quill, Arnold and Back 2009; Schofield et al. 2006; Waldrop and Rinfrette 2009). Each of these considerations contributes to an often highly charged and complex interpersonal dynamic (Heedman and Starkhammar 2002; Johnson et al. 2011).

In such situations, emotions and interpersonal subjectivities may influence doctors' approaches and decisions within patient care (Brickner et al. 2004). Subjective influences may subtly shape the timing of treatment decisions, the choices made, pathways taken and care experiences. This does not sit well with the notion of the distanced, dispassionate medical practitioner making decisions on the basis of objective benefit and quality of life (Nettleton, Burrows and Watt 2008). Nevertheless, as shown in the interview excerpts I present below, subjective influences are evident within doctors' accounts of their everyday medical work. Emotion matters as a *skill*; conversations about dying, palliation and the end of life demand a careful balance of empathy, kindness and separateness. A clinician's capacity to 'do' emotions (whether dissociation, empathy, sympathy, withdrawal, and so on) is critical to professional 'competence' and 'expertise' irrespective of how these are defined. Few researchers have explored how doctors themselves experience and interpret this complex process, a gap I seek to address here.

## Into the Field

### *When to Talk About Dying and the Shift to Palliative and End-of-life Care?*

As outlined in Chapter 1, in this Chapter I draw on a series of interviews conducted in late 2011 and early 2012 with senior Australian doctors located in hospitals in Queensland (i.e. staff specialists), with between 16 and 30 years in medical practice (YIMP). I focused on those regularly referring patients for palliative and/or end-of-life care over the past 12 months. Over 80 per cent of referrals to the specialist palliative care in Australia are cancer related, and thus cancer-related medical specialties make up a significant proportion of the sample. The senior doctors interviewed come from a range of medical specialties including medical oncology, haematology, surgery, radiation oncology, general medicine, palliative care and geriatrics. What connects them for this study is that they are each required to initiate discussions about futility, the lack of meaningful curative interventions and, ultimately, the need for specialist palliative care. The interviews began with discussion around their perceptions in terms of *how* and *when* to broach the subject of palliative care and end-of-life issues. They had varied approaches and I provide a series of indicative responses:

> *Interviewer*: ... at what point do you talk about dying?
>
> *Specialist* (male): I would talk about prognosis, ah, so living is the emphasis, more than dying. From the initiation of the association [therapeutic relationship] … you start to say, "Look this is something that is not going to be curable, this is something that we can control and eke out a little bit", and talk about average times, and what might happen ... So I guess it's when I start to see physiology, that indicates to me that the wheels are falling off ... then you start to say, "Well, this is not going the right way." [Urology, YIMP: 23, private]

Another participant comments:

> *Specialist* (female): …You shouldn't be having that discussion [of being terminal] when you're sending them to palliative care ... where they get more of a shock, is where they don't see things as deteriorating, whereas you do. So, that's more what sometimes generates the angst. I see the patients deteriorating and the patient doesn't see it, or the family don't want to see it, do you know what I

> mean? … [But] you should've already had the discussion about your intent of treatment, well before that point. [Medical Oncology, YIMP: 19, public]

Another participant comments:

> *Specialist* (male): And I think as a principle [talking about palliation] is a good thing, but the difficulty I find is actually trying to put that into the initial conversation ... And so I think it's very difficult for the patient sometimes because they have a preconceived idea that palliative care means doing nothing you know, that you've given up, that you're not giving it a go, or you're not having active treatment ... So I think it's difficult, even though you try and order things so you get the palliative care referral in early, I think a lot of the time the patients don't really want to, they don't want to go there. That of course could be a problem with how we're presenting it. [Medical Oncology, YIMP: 23, public and private]

The initial conversation within the interviews about discussing the end of life revealed a broad consensus around the importance of 'bringing it [referral] up early' but frustration with the perceived practical limitations in achieving this. They consistently talked about the importance of early discussions about potential terminality and unanimously supported a policy of disclosing this to patients very early on. Yet, this was also viewed as problematic, and sometimes impossible, due to a perceived 'resistance' or 'denial' on the part of their patients and their families, and the lack of resources committed to palliative care within their respective institutional contexts. A revealing aspect of the interviews – and perhaps more critical than their literal responses – was the frequency of conversational turns and emphases evident when the specialists' were asked about their own experiences of referral. As shown above, and in the majority of the other interviews, while the participants were each asked specifically how *they felt* about and approached discussions about palliative care, they tended to divert the discussion away from them and towards *the patient* (that is, about patient angst or emotional difficulty). Such conversational tactics reveal the very challenge of acknowledging their own difficulties around discussions about the end of life and the referral process. This includes tensions around normative understandings about how a 'good doctor' should be (that is, caring yet detached, emotional yet objective). What emerges is a narrative across the interviewees' accounts that suggest a fusion between specialist and patient subjectivities and forms of emotion.

## *The Art of Referring and the Importance of Representation*

A key theme within the interviews was the rhetorical and interactional strategies that were deemed necessary to manage dialogue about terminality and the end of life. One should not underestimate the intense difficulty of many conversations about the futility of further treatment and the end of life for patients, family and clinicians. Such discussions may be the first time that the person has heard that there is no longer any hope for long-term survival, presenting significant existential and interpersonal dilemmas. I was interested in how these specialists accounted for the emotionality of such interactions and the strategies they used to deliver difficult and challenging news to their patients:

> *Specialist* (female): ... I sell them [palliative care] as being whiz-bang at helping with symptoms, and accessible, and I say, "You might not need them now, but if you've met them, if you need them in the future, it's easy to ring them". And I don't have anyone really who recoils in horror, and refuses. [Radiation Oncology, YIMP: 26, public]

Another participant comments:

> *Specialist* (male): Um, and I tend to be pretty proactive about it … I try and pre-empt them and say, "Look, you know, the thing is, you're probably going to die at some stage. It's not going to happen right now but I'd very much prefer if you met the palliative care colleagues, so you get to know a friendly face", and you're not you know, half-dead... [Surgery, YIMP: 16, public]

A significant hurdle from the specialists' perspectives was the stigma associated with moving to specialist palliative care and attempting to communicate the need for such a transition without reflecting a sense of hopelessness or that they were 'giving up' on their patient. Most explained how they developed 'up-beat' rhetorical strategies to present palliative care clinicians to patients and family as benevolent, friendly, highly skilled and 'not needed yet'. One specialist talked about how he just 'sort of play[s] it dumb' and states, 'I'm just the surgeon', when confronted with the issue of palliative care. In fact, most viewed telling patients early on as easier (for them) in that they could remain positive and relaxed and as one participant stated, say things like, 'You're not dying yet, but do me a favour and meet with them'. This allowed them to diffuse potential emotional responses in facing imminent mortality while moving toward a model of shared care. The participants focused on the importance of the rhetorical presentation of palliation and of utilising 'softer terminology' to not emphasise terminality and the end of life. The use of certain framings and words was viewed as critical to how patients and families might respond:

> *Specialist* (male): ... We'll call it supportive care, but that's another sort of term I've learned recently is a good one, because, and ah, almost a time to say, "Look it's now … it's about all of them, and it's, and you know it's, it's supportive

> to help you out when we can't really do anything about this now, these are the folk that look after you". ... [When you say this] you know they going to die, they know they're going to die, but you feel terrible! ... So I still make an appointment [in three months], even though sometimes you know they won't even be back for that ... you're giving them some little bit of hope ... [Surgery, YIMP: 16, public]

Another participant comments:

> *Specialist* (male): But you see, palliative care is terminal, "I'm about to die," rather than incurable which is a very open-ended word. [Incurable] allows you to sort of construct your life, or construct your circumstances according to your personality, beliefs, attitudes, all those sorts of things. So that's the problem with the connotation, that it's perceived as "I'm about to die, nothing can be done." [Medical Oncology, YIMP: 40, private]

The participants each offered accounts of the importance of the specific wording and strategies of representation in discussions about the need for the movement to specialist palliative care. Each talked of developing strategies for 'making it easier on patients', including proposing future follow-up appointments they knew would not be kept. It was clear that these rhetorical and organisational strategies were about making it emotionally easier for them as well as their patients, reframing palliative care as 'advanced', 'well resourced' and 'highly skilled' rather than indicative of the end of life. The effect was to reduce the potential for an immediate crisis response from their patients, which was presented as a challenging interpersonal dynamic. While potentially problematic (see Smith et al. 2010 on honesty and hope), what lies at the core of these specialists' accounts is how *they feel* about communicating about terminality, mortality and the loss of more 'active' treatment options. In the following section I focus on this particular issue – how the interviewees, as doctors, account for their own feelings in such contexts.

## *Specialists' Accounts of Emotions in Referral to Palliative Care*

The interviews provided the opportunity to ask the specialists not merely about the logics underpinning their referral practices but also how referring felt to them. While emotions are reflected in all aspects of their accounts to some degree, I was interested in their explicit reflections on emotion. I treat these accounts as both *genuine reflections* of emotion as experienced, and as forms of *impression management*. They are self-representations of recalled emotional responses, reflecting dynamics between the researcher and the participant (cf. Nettleton, Burrows and Watt 2008), and normative discourses around 'good doctoring':

> *Specialist* (male): ... No, I don't find it [referral to palliative care] hard. It's not that there's no emotion attached to it, there isn't a lot of emotion attached to it, you do what you can, and then move onto the next person … you may argue that I do it well or badly, but I've been doing it for as long as I do, with respect, because the people [doctors] who really care, don't last, because it's too, you know, to actually carry that emotional baggage with you, you're not going to sustain yourself … [Medical Oncology, YIMP: 40, private]

Another participant comments:

> *Specialist* (male): ... probably we tend to avoid the really difficult [end of life] issues, and sort of hope that the palliative care physician will deal with those things. Because, I mean, I personally find those end of life kind of issues very difficult to deal with, and to broach with a patient. [Surgery, YIMP: 21, public and private]

Another participant comments:

> *Specialist* (male): … you get into a model of pragmatism about pointing out what is and is not possible for them. Um, relating empathically with them about that, and sometimes those are difficult conversations, sometimes they last longer than you would like ... [Urology, YIMP: 23, private]

Another participant comments:

> *Specialist* (male): … I do take the emotion out of it, and it's very factual. I don't know if that's offensive to people, but that's just the way I do it ... if you get overly involved emotionally, you're not going to give necessarily the best care, because your inside, or your decision-making process is blurred. So, you can still feel for people, but at the end of the day, yeah, you're not overly involved emotionally ... I stopped going to funerals a long time ago … [Haematology, YIMP: 25, private]

Talk of emotion was highly varied, with each grappling with how to process the potentially emotional aspects of their work. They would talk about 'a model of pragmatism', 'tak[ing] the emotion out of it', and being unable to 'really care', as well as the problems associated with colleagues who could not achieve this (I explore this in more detail below). These, and the other participants' accounts, reveal dissociative strategies utilised in everyday clinical work to minimise the perceived impacts of emotion; unconscious strategies, some would argue, to avoid the potential for 'compassion fatigue' (see Najjar et al. 2009) and enable the articulation of 'detached concern' (Fox and Lief 1963; see also Fox 2006). Not getting involved emotionally was viewed as an important skill to develop in order to avoid 'burning out'. Some degree of emotional withdrawal was interlinked with professionalism and competent doctoring, with control of empathy being viewed as expertise. Yet, there was also awareness of the limits of dissociation and the importance of sentimentality in being a competent doctor:

> *Specialist* (male): I mean emotionally it can be difficult, and the point of view that I'm cutting myself off ... well, I think that's a bit of a cop out. And in fact the point in time when I do that, is going to be the time when you're really missing out on something. Because even though it might be emotionally draining, if you just stand back and say, "Well, here you go, on your way", that's a problem, I think, well, you might say that you're protecting yourself, but in fact you're missing out on some [thing] ... that's not a very healthy approach, not to get involved [Medical Oncology, YIMP: 23, public and private]

Even within this group of specialists there was a wide range of self-reported emotional responses to discussions around referral to specialist palliative care. There were those who talked about being affected but resilient (the majority), as well as those who insisted that they were unaffected by emotions (the minority). There were also those who talked about the day-to-day emotional effects of talking about death and dying:

> *Specialist* (male): ... you do think, "Okay, he's about my age", or "He's got kids around my age", you know. I've got a number of young women, who had bad disease, and they've got little kids, and you feel for them, you really feel for them … sometimes you'll just have one of those bad days where I come out of here thinking, "Oh Christ, how many people have I told they're going to die today" ... [Surgery, YIMP: 33, private]

Another participant comments:

> *Specialist* (female): For the ones that, you know, they've been your patient [for a while], but you just have to say goodbye. I think you go ahead and, it's almost like you deliver it, and then you know, I'll probably be low for maybe the next 15, 20 minutes. But then, to be very honest, you have to see the next patient that's actually waiting to see you outside. [Medical Oncology, YIMP: 18, public]

While it was clear that such conversations and negotiations around referral had emotional impacts on the participants, these were articulated as 'fleeting' and 'temporary'. The broader cultural acceptability of emotional talk within the workplace is also important to consider here, in particular, norms of everyday emotional talk within the medical profession and their organisations. It was revealing that the participants talked about having little sense of what other doctors felt regarding 'letting patients go' and the lack of reported 'emotion talk' in day-to-day interactions:

> *Interviewer*: How do you see your colleagues dealing with these conversations [about end of life]?
>
> *Specialist* (male): I've no idea, because we don't often talk about it. So because in fact in medical oncology we're treaters, if you know what I mean? We have treatment options, people come to us and say, "What drug can you give me?" So we operate out of a different framework. So, do we sit down over a few drinks and talk about that [end of life discussions]? No. What do we talk about? Clinical trials, latest treatments you know, how does it apply to these patients? They're the conversations that we have ... [Medical Oncology, YIMP: 42, private]

Most professional groups do not systematically reflect collectively on the emotional character of their work. I do not present these accounts as reflective of professional pathology; rather, as a reflection of potential norms evident within some biomedical contexts that may shape the validity of emotion and thus how it is managed within clinical settings. Another consequence talked about in the interviews was the tendency to maintain an emphasis on potentially 'life prolonging' options and the role of emotion therein.

### *Prolonging Life, Emotion and the Role of Ego*

An important theme within the interviews was the observed potential for a part emotional and part ego driven form of *medical activism* in pre palliative care contexts. This was talked about as problematic but also 'natural' given doctor and patient desire for life-prolonging intervention. A 'treat till the death' narrative was evident across the participants' accounts, articulated as embedded in a curative and disease (rather than person) focus of biomedicine:

> *Specialist* (male): There are some doctors who don't necessarily see the patient, they see the disease, and it's a personal battle against the disease. And I think it's a maturity thing, where you get beyond that in your practice, but some people don't ... it's a battle against the disease, and they're always coming up with something else, and the patient's a side piece to it ... And whether that causes a reluctance to let go, or whether it's a reluctance to be let go, I think is probably hard to define, and I think it's a bit of both ... [Haematology, YIMP: 25, private]

Another participant comments:

> *Specialist* (male): … "We've got something for you!" … We go, "Here's a trial, you could go on this?" And they go, "Well, this must be good you know, if it's a trial it's something fantastic." Even though you could go to great lengths to say, "This is not going to cure your lung cancer," people often have unrealistic expectations … [Medical Oncology, YIMP: 23, public and private]

Another participant comments:

> *Specialist* (male): I suppose initially [the need for palliation] it's just the admission that we've been defeated by the disease. [Surgery, YIMP: 21, public and private]

Another participant comments:

> *Specialist* (male): Often it is a personal [doctor's] battle against cancer and that's hard to let go of for some of us I think [Medical Oncology, YIMP: 25, public]

The above excerpts capture the participants' concerns about the assumptive basis of much clinical practice; a focus on, as another specialist stated, 'beating it or nothing'. Yet, the picture was much more complex with the specialists often talking about the significant and sustained pressure from patients and families as driving the pursuit of 'active' treatment:

> *Specialist* (male): I don't think I'm probably as, probably not referring people as early as I should, I'm sure most people would probably willingly accept that that's the case.
>
> *Interviewer*: Why?
>
> *Specialist*: Again because of that issue; largely because they come for treatment, and a lot of the time they're not willing to accept that they, that they're not going to have active treatment ... [Medical Oncology, YIMP: 23, public and private]

Another participant comments:

> *Specialist* (male): But there are some people that will be absolutely determined to go down in flames, and you cannot do anything about that, that is the way, that to them is the only acceptable way to die, not giving up. And you can explain to them that "you're going to get sick, it's very unlikely that you're going to get any benefit. If you do get a benefit in terms of remission, it's going to be very brief," and they will still want to have more treatment ... [Haematology, YIMP: 25, private]

The interviews revealed a precarious situation with overtreatment often viewed as an outcome of collusion on the part of the doctor and patient. All parties to some extent were presented as reluctant to cease active treatment. The 'dogged pursuit of active treatment', as one doctor described it, was talked about as underpinned by a subjective perception of the medical role as 'disease beater' rather than bearer of 'bad news'. Viewed as part ego and part biomedical culture, such a position was considered as having some influence on patient pathways to palliation. This was captured in one participant's statement that many doctors 'want to make a mark by getting a survival response'. In this way the interviews provided significant insight into the *potential* (albeit varying) influences of ego, emotion and the inter-subjective in shaping care trajectories. Much of this variability was also talked about as embedded in training in emotion management (or lack thereof).

### Training for (and Doing) Emotion

Across the participants' accounts there was considerable concern regarding the ways in which the skills of balancing objectivity and empathy, and concern versus detachment, were learnt or taught. Each acknowledged the emotional management and maturity necessary to have 'successful conversations' with patients about mortality, while suggesting that for doctors a proneness to emotion was unsustainable. A certain degree of dissociation was critical to their profession. Talking to patients about dying, as articulated by the participants, was often viewed as 'hit and miss' and a process of 'learning from mistakes'.

> *Interviewer*: How do you teach talking about dying?
>
> *Specialist* (female): Um, I think the registrars just need to learn by watching us do it, year in and year out … They need to learn language … that is sensible and conveys some degree of regret, some degree of empathy, but they also have to not be too emotive in their own reactions to it, you know … [junior doctors] they burn out if they get too involved … you sort of learn over the years what works and what doesn't. [Medical Oncology, YIMP: 19, public]

Another participant comments:

> *Specialist* (male): I don't think we're well trained in knowing how to broach those subjects in a sensitive manner, and generally, I mean, we're sort of taught to always give patients hope, and once you get to that stage you know where you have to admit that there is no longer any hope, I think that is a really hard thing to admit. [Surgery, YIMP: 21, public and private]

Another participant comments:

> *Specialist* (male): ... it still comes down to people, based on personalities … some people are just still not cut out for these jobs. And trying to stop people going down that route is darn hard! And there's no way in the system that actually stops you doing that sometimes. You try not to have people who you don't think are going to cope with some of these things [the end of life] upfront. But once they're travelling down this pathway, trying to get them off it, is nigh on impossible. [Medical Oncology, YIMP: 32, public and private]

It was revealing in the interviews that emotions were constructed as necessary for good doctoring but that there was little or no training or mentoring in how to talk about emotions or talk about death. Appropriate strategies had to be 'learnt on the job'. The expectation that junior doctors in particular be sensitive yet distanced without significant training in communication was viewed as particularly problematic and was talked about as leading those clinicians who were 'overly emotional' to the point of burnout. Such accounts highlight not only the subjectivities of talk about dying and palliative care, but also the ways biomedical culture perpetuates or encourages certain ways of being with, and talking with, patients about particular issues.

## Discussion

I have started this book with a focus on the perspective of doctors, which may seem curious for some readers. My reason for this point of departure is that doctors remain key to the timely topicalisation of, and recognition of, the dying process. Moreover, how they manage such challenging and emotive discussions contributes to (or not, as the case may be) the broader de-stigmatisation of the dying process for individuals and their families. Yet, as can be seen in the interviews, many doctors find the fact that their patients are dying highly problematic, themselves holding onto hope for longevity, and even continuing futile treatments (or those only 'technically' life-prolonging). When accompanied by lack of recognition of the negotiation of dying as *art, subjective* and *relational*, the potential for problems in clinical contexts is significant. Given that the very construction and definition of dying remains highly dependent on expert engagement and clinical judgement, I viewed it as pertinent to begin the book with an exploration of medical accounts of emotions-at-work and to provide a critical examination of their reflective capacity as mediators of futility and dying – and to unpack their broader (dis)comforts with managing transitions to the end of life. As indicated, Chapters 3, 4 and 5 focus in on patient experiences and provide an important source of comparison to the accounts presented in this chapter. While throughout this book I emphasise that dying is a physiological and embodied event, I argue that it is also heavily shaped by the lay–professional interface, the character of medical expertise, and the capacity of biomedicine to understand its own therapeutic limits and the implications of its ambitions. Dying, as emphasised in more detail in subsequent chapters, is morally laden and cultural produced, with the co-production of death denial or resistance to death by patient *and* doctor a critical, persistent and problematic dynamic.

Returning to the specificities of the results presented above, it is not new to emphasise the subjective and emotional underpinnings of medical work. This area has received considerable attention from sociologists over the past 50 years (Fox 1959, Fox and Lief 1963; James 1989; Strauss et al. 1982). Scholars have situated medical work within a dialectic of individualism (autonomy, subjectivity, experience) vis-à-vis professional control (rationality, regulation and systematisation) (Freidson 1988). Within this scholarly tradition, questions around emotion, subjectivity and forms of sentimentality have been explored (Lupton 1997; Nettleton, Burrows and Watt 2008; Strauss et al. 1982; Wallace and Lemaire 2007), including in end-of-life contexts (Christakis 1999; Fox 2006), but hitherto not in the context of the practice of referral to palliative and end-of-life care and discussions about dying. I have attempted to unpack recognition of dying and referral to palliative care as embedded in subjective experience, emotions and the priorities and ideologies espoused in current biomedical culture.

The interviews with clinicians revealed several important themes related to topicalising dying and the need for a transition to palliative and/or end-of-life care, and the strategic representation of this transition. This process emerged as being deeply entrenched in the specialists' own preferences for particular forms of interaction and interpersonal dynamics. Their accounts illustrate significant self-reported difficulties in raising the issue of palliation and dying with patients and the need for the development of rhetorical tactics and interpersonal strategies for 'easing patients into it' and dealing with 'patients who are in denial' (see also Brown et al. 2009; Friedrichsen and Strang 2003). Strategic representations were common including 'toning down' talk of mortality and dying and focusing on the finer competencies of palliative care teams, such as them having more relevant expertise, practitioner benevolence and enhanced resources. While much emphasis was placed on the emotional difficulties for their patients and how to *manage these* within the clinical encounter, it was clear within their accounts that such tactics revealed much about their own emotions and interactional preferences. The interviews provided an opportunity to explore how referral may be mediated by the specialists' individual desires, subjective experiences and emotional characteristics.

A second major theme to emerge from the interviews was in the participants' accounts of emotions and subjectivity in their experiences of discussions about palliation and the end of life. The discussions were a difficult task in some respects. In the interviews the participants' often shifted the focus of analysis away from their own emotions, and onto those of their patients, revealing a reluctance to engage with their *own* feelings (cf. Nettleton, Burrows and Watt 2008). Although they talked about how referring patients feels, this talk was often formulaic. They discussed displaying empathy but simultaneously offered evidence of detached concern (Fox and Lief 1963; see also Fox 2006). They used the term empathy, and offered experiential accounts of *being* empathetic, yet there was often little evidence of emotional engagement as opposed to the performance of emotion (cf. Graham 2006). One explanation is that the presentation of detached concern allows for the avoidance of experienced or imagined 'compassion fatigue' (Najjar et al. 2009) while retaining an expert, professional character; displaying concern and superficial empathy, but remaining objective.

Such representations of *workable* displays of emotion also relate to normative modes of clinician behaviour, particularly in terms of the medico-cultural validity of public displays of emotion. For example, being 'overly emotional' was negatively connoted by the majority of participants, and was associated with a lack of professionalism, a lack of expertise, or a weakness of strength of character. The frequent examples of colleagues who had 'burnt out' or 'couldn't cope' due to being 'too emotionally involved' was a clear indication of this. In this way we see delineation between the perceived benefits of emotional engagement and the performance of emotion. Displaying measured pre-determined empathy was more beneficial for the specialist than genuine emotional engagement. This is not to say that the doctors I interviewed were disingenuous, rather, that they clearly understood the benefits of performing emotional work and the potential pitfalls of 'caring too much'.

Other research has documented the ambivalence of doctors towards emotion and subjectivity within clinical decision making and my research complements this. As Nettleton, Burrows and Watt (2008: 18) observed regarding NHS doctors' emotion:

> The feelings they articulate are riven with ambivalence. We suggest that this is generated by a contextual tension which presumes that the medical profession are required to reproduce medicine as an abstract system – an objective, trustworthy, reliable, effective, competent and fair mode of healing – and yet individual practitioners are also required to be caring, emotionally intelligent, intuitive, and sensitive.

Indeed, the degree of distress that could and would be involved in being emotionally engaged with each terminal 'dying' patient would likely be intolerable within these clinical contexts. As Nettleton, Burrows and Watt (2008) argue, clinicians expect to strike a consistent balance between the rational and the emotional self. Yet, even in simulated contexts, doctors show high stress responses to breaking bad news and discussions about terminality (Brown et al. 2009). Consistent with Nettleton, Burrows and Watt (2008), this chapter shows the ambiguity of emotion management within the broader habitus of medical culture: the ideal type of doctor who manages perfectly the precarious balance between professionalism and emotionality; the doctor who maintains a focus on empathising with a patient in order to add therapeutic value to the treatment experience while simultaneously maintaining the necessary level of detachment or dissociation.

Such expectations are clearly unrealistic, particularly given the participants' reflections on 'burnout' and the clear lack of formalised training on the emotional character of death and dying talk. Acknowledgment of futility and dying is not compromised by human subjective influences, but it is important to explore and capture such inter-subjective influences. On a broader level, the doctors' accounts question the challenges and ambivalences of contemporary medical work and the need to reproduce medicine as an abstract system (Nettleton, Burrows and Watt 2008) imbued with objectivity and distance, whilst retaining the emotionality of the relationship and event. To imagine faith/hope/intuition and rationality/objectivity to sit comfortably together is an unrealistic expectation of medicine and its practitioners. A number of the participants did recount growing less emotionally involved as they continued their careers. In sum, this chapter reveals the ways in which clinicians struggle with the questions of hope and futility, illustrating that decisions about topicalising futility, acknowledgment of dying and the referral to palliative care are as much an art as a science.

Doctors' accounts provide a situated and partial viewing of the transition to, and experience of, palliative and end-of-life care. As outlined in the introduction, these processes are multi-stakeholder and intersubjective, with patients, families and nurses in turn contributing in important ways. Thus, the following chapters explore the accounts of people/patients who have themselves made the transition to end-of-life care, providing important insights into the lived experience of such transitions and the dying process. This takes the form of a person-centred understanding of how many of the discontents outlined above (and others), can manifest within individual accounts of illness, dying and care. Moreover, in Chapters 5 and 6 I augment these accounts through an examination of other stakeholder perspectives and roles including those of nurses and families, working towards a multi-stakeholder and rounded understanding of dying as a social occasion.

# Chapter 3
# A Place for Dying

## Introduction

There have been some significant professional and organisational shifts in the delivery of care for the dying over the course of the twentieth, and now twenty-first centuries. These new sites of care for the dying – namely in-patient hospices and specialist palliative care units – represent major shifts in how dying is done. As outlined in the Introduction, for the majority of the history of humanity, dying has taken place in the home (Howarth 2007a). The increased availability of 'institutions for dying' has begun to subtly shift the way some people and their carers experience the dying process (Thomas, Morris and Clark 2004), shifting the roles, responsibilities and overall 'burden' of caring for the dying (James, and Field 1992; Kellehear 2007; Lawton 1998, 2000; Li 2004; Li and Arber 2006; McNamara 2004). This relocation of much dying to institutions has raised important questions around the implications of shifts in *places for dying*. In Australia relatively few people now die at home (around 16 per cent), with over 20 per cent dying in hospices, 10 per cent in nursing homes and the remaining dying in hospitals (Department of Health 2010). Yet, little research has been completed on the lived experience of dying in a hospice or specialist palliative care unit despite it becoming a more common place for dying (for an exception see Lawton 2000).

In this chapter I focus on developing a critical sociology of the hospice as concurrently enabling but also significantly disabling in certain situations. I explore the tensions and complexities people can experience when entering the hospice environment to die, situating my analysis within broader sociological concerns around the medicalisation and sequestration of dying as manifest in the hospice movement (James and Field 1992; Howarth 2007a; Lawton 1998, 2000). Moreover, I focus on how the *place of dying* fundamentally shapes the dying process and lived experiences at the end of life. As highlighted in the accounts of in-patients, hospices limit and allow certain things (for discussions around religiosity and assisting dying see Chapter 4). In this way I argue that the hospice comes with a set of (evolving) *normative moralities* but also *liberating possibilities.* And moreover, that these have significant implications for how people die and forms of dying privileged within this context. Some reflection on the existing literature exploring the institutional inflection of dying is useful to provide a platform for discussion of the outcomes of my fieldwork in a hospice.

## Background

### *The (Gradual) Shift of Dying to Institutions*

Prior to the twentieth century, hospitals were significantly limited in their capacity to provide relief at the end of life (Howarth 2007a: 117). However, through processes of professionalisation and institutionalisation – including increased public health services and expanded health resources – dying *in an institution* became a more viable option in many countries. As Howarth (2007a) argues, and as I discussed previously in the Introduction, this fundamentally altered the experience and character of dying and continues to heavily inflect individual experiences at the end of life. The development of care for the dying as a specialised medical practice thus promoted the relocation of much death and dying to institutions (Clark 2007).

Such shifts were not merely about expertise, resources and technology; rather, they reflected important social and cultural changes around gender roles and the structure of family life (see also Chapter 5). Specifically, as Howarth (2007a: 117) argues, a key influence on the shift toward institutional dying was the increased participation of women in the workforce and their reduced capacity to provide care in the home at the end of life. This gendered sociocultural shift, among other influences, encouraged the state (via public healthcare delivery) to take a greater role in care of the dying. The expansionist tendencies within biomedicine – including the desire to extend formalised, specialised biomedical care to end-of-life contexts (that is, development of palliative and hospice as 'medical' expertise) – interplayed with cultural shifts around care, responsibility and increasing reliance on the state. These dynamics may shift again with retracting willingness of many OECD countries to deliver such comprehensive public healthcare, including care of the dying, under conditions of economic constraint. However, hospice and specialised in-patient palliative care services continue to prosper and expand, requiring, in my mind, significant sociological investigation.

The major developments over of the twentieth century in care for the dying saw significant improvements in support, including more systematic control over pain and physiological suffering, but in turn raised important questions around the extent to which dying could be managed as a clinical problem (see Introduction for more extended discussion). This included dilemmas around the interplay of professional care *with* such things as ritual, belief, spirituality, ethics and moralities (Broom 2012b): how to systematise the care of the dying and manage bioethical considerations, given individual beliefs and the need to acknowledge and embrace cultural values and practices. The rise of 'the institution' provided a particular type of 'solution' (Howarth 2007b), often raising new and significant normative or reductive problems (cf. Foucault 1977).

Significant criticisms quickly emerged around the limits of medicine to adequately deal with dying outside the home (Illick 1976; James and Field 1992) and the threat of institutions providing inadequate, restrictive and alienating care at the end of life (Howarth 2007a: 117). Herein lay a major challenge for the hospice or hospital death: avoiding the significant potential for a sequestration of dying (Lawton 1998). The hospice movement sought, in some respects, to counter this potential by focusing on the development of an institutional form of care that was firmly centred on amelioration of suffering, holistic care and psychosocial support, that is, instead of a focus on intervention and life-prolongment, focusing on life-enhancement. While this set of ideals offered a new way of doing dying in an institutional form (cf. Bradshaw 1996), hospices and palliative care services quickly came under criticism for reductive or medicalised understandings of 'dying well'. They functioned to both separate dying from normal life (sequester) and to institutionalise (medicalise) it. Notions of good deaths circulated within the milieu, contributing to the development of a new institutional and professionally-espoused normativity around death and dying.

It is not that hospital-based or hospice-based deaths are necessarily problematic. On the contrary, there was (and continues to be) a significant need for state and professional support for dying beyond the home. Rather, the process of institutionalisation brought with it the prioritisation of certain ways of doing dying and value being placed on certain approaches to death. As suggested by Howarth (2007a: 121), the doctor replaced the priest at the deathbed, and the hospice or specialist palliative care unit is increasingly replacing the home. Rather than a focus on the afterlife or preparation for 'what follows', the emphasis came to be placed on pain relief and symptom control or amelioration. Technology and professional power thus interplayed to shift the balance of power and the locus of control away from the patient and families, to the professional and profession (and institution) (Howarth 2007a: 123). In this sense, *place* in the context of dying has become much more than a matter of location, aesthetics, bonds and comforts of home. Rather, it is about control, power and choices at the end of life. The location of dying and the movement toward institutional deaths shifted power and also decreased visibility.

Lawton (1998) provided a rather stark analysis of this potential, with an ethnographic study of the sequestering of dying and the potentially sequestered character of hospice deaths, with the institution facilitating professional control of what were previously 'natural ends' and in turn protecting society from our dirty and destabilising ends. The horror of dying (cf. Kristeva 1982) and the potential community visibility of home deaths thus make the shift toward intuitional dying a socially important shift and one with significant implications. Glaser and Strauss (1968) were among the early sociologists to emphasise the problematic shift of dying in the hospital and the implications therein. While in many respects the hospice movement reflects a degree of resistance to the medicalisation of death (Howarth 2007a: 123), it still offers an institutional inflection point of dying, offering new and important dilemmas to patients, families and health professionals.

### *Understanding the Hospice Experience*

As a place for dying, hospice and specialist in-patient palliative care is constantly evolving and has many forms across different countries and cultural contexts. Despite representing a major shift in how we do death, relatively little research has been completed on hospice deaths (e.g. Bradshaw 1996; Hart, Sainsbury and Short 1998; Howarth 2007b; Lawton 1998, 2000; McNamara, Waddell and Colvin 1995). The hospice offers not only a unique place for dying but also a unique philosophy of care and dying. Largely founded on Christian values and beliefs, the hospice movement has evolved into twenty-first century to incorporate various aspects of medical as well as social and cultural values (Howarth 2007a: 139). Seeking to provide relief from 'total pain', the hospice has been criticised for extending the medical control of dying to incorporate a much broader series of issues beyond symptom control and alleviation. Part of a recognised problematic of the hospice model and experience is the issue of control and particularly medical control (Howarth 2007a: 139). In-patient hospice medicine has evolved significantly over the last few decades, raising significant questions and controversy regarding deviations from the original hospice ethos and around the emerging 'hierarchies of care' in an increasingly biomedicalised environment (James and Field 1992). While views differ on the veracity of such claims and the value of contemporary forms of hospice care, there is little doubt that medico-cultural shifts in the institutionalised forms of dying warrant investigation (Broom and Tovey 2007a; Howarth 2007b). Yet, there have been relatively few attempts to systematically examine hospice experiences, largely due to the difficulties of researching the end of life.

In considering places for dying, it is worth considering the resonance of contemporary patient preferences and choices. What do people actually want at the end of life? Do their desires shift over time and in the last few weeks? Are they able to achieve these preferences? The assumption in the biomedical literature has often been that patients want to die at home (Higginson and Sen-Gupta 2000), yet this is being debunked by recent research that indicates a much stronger preference for death in a hospice or specialist palliative care unit than previously indicated (Thomas, Morris and Clark 2004). Yet, little qualitative work has been done tracing the broader experience of those in contemporary in-patient hospice care (see Cannaerts, Dierckx de Casterlé and Grypdonck 2004; Lawton 1998; McPherson, Wilson and Murray 2007). Drawing on the experiences of people in the last few weeks of life, in this chapter I explore the difficulties, pleasures and tensions evident in this critical juncture between life and death.

### *The Enactment of Dying and Dying in an Institution*

Notions of 'the good death' permeate the sociological and biomedical literature on death and dying (see Hart, Sainsbury and Short 1998). While often referring to an ideal to be achieved, the 'good death' also represents a sociological critique of overly prescriptive notions of appropriate behaviours in and around dying (Howarth 2007b: 132). While not wanting to overemphasise the constructed character of the end of life, it is worth noting that research has illustrated some performative elements of dying, including the expectations and structures surrounding patient–patient and patient–clinician interactions. Sontag (1991) and Seale (2001) have emphasised the discursive and rhetorical practices often utilised by clinicians, carers and other stakeholders ('be strong' or 'fight hard') and potential impacts on patient wellbeing. Similarly, the characterisation of patients as 'difficult', 'a problem' or 'loved' has been shown to operate in healthcare contexts, and there exists potential for individuals to be disciplined for transgressing 'appropriate' patient roles (see also Li and Arber 2006). Here lies the performative aspect of dying: the ways in which certain ways of being (and dying) are allowed, encouraged, accepted or marginalised (Howarth 2007b). While there has been some work done on how talk between hospice clinicians perpetuates such understandings (Li and Arber 2006), little work has been done on patient accounts of the performativity of 'an accomplished death'. As such, I explore patient accounts of suppressing or utilising certain forms of action, talk or expression in the in-patient hospice context.

### *What the Hospice Environment 'Does' to Dying*

The hospice environment, and its various permutations, has received both admiration and criticism from social scientists. For example, the notion of the sanitisation of death and dying has emerged consistently within the social science literature, with various critiques around the perceived routinisation, medicalisation and bureaucratisation of death and dying (Bradshaw 1996; Howarth 2007b). James and Field (1992) argued that routinisation and pressures toward bureaucratisation and professionalisation have fundamentally shifted the character of hospice care. While such criticisms are disputed by many of those working in palliative care and in-patient hospice settings, what is clear is that the in-patient hospice environment is unique and evolving and that it presents certain constraints as well as possibilities (Howarth 2007b; Lawton 2000). I take a phenomenological focus, approaching the hospice as a space that is experienced in certain ways and that allows or promotes certain experiences or emotions. I argue that the hospice allows possibilities, such as hope, play and a space for living, but also presents unique challenges to the individual, such as liminal spheres and pressure to be 'accomplished' in the dying process (Froggatt 1997; Little et al. 1998; Navona and Morag 2004). A focus on these micro-level experiences, including their importance for interpersonal authenticity and recognition at the end of life, is critical for developing a better sociological understanding of the hospice in-patient experience.

## Into the Field

### *Expectations and Understandings of Hospice Care*

The interviews I draw on here were completed with in-patients who were in the last few weeks of life and receiving care in a hospice in New South Wales, Australia. The hospice was established in 1993 and offers a twenty-bed in-patient facility for people close to the end of life. It, and the hospital it is part of, is owned by a Catholic organisation that owns and runs hospitals and healthcare services in several locations throughout Australia. This organisation was one of the first Catholic entities established in colonial Australia. It is funded through a combination of private and public funds with an agreement with the local health authority to deliver certain health services. This funding arrangement gives more control to the organisation in terms of trajectory and representation, than in the case of purely State-funded organisations. This history and connectivity to the Catholic Church in all likelihood enhances the organisation's sensitivities towards, and willingness to promote, specific Christian values around death and dying. In saying this, referrals to the hospice come from throughout the region and the hospice is not promoted as a Christian service, but rather, an end-of-life care service. As such, the following data (and that used in subsequent chapters which draw on hospice-based data) should be viewed as specific to this hospice but also touching on important themes likely relevant to other in-patient hospice care facilities in Australia and internationally.

In the interviews I focused on the participants' expectations of dying in a hospice, with a particular emphasis on *place* for dying and experiences of transitioning to the hospice. Although the interviews took place when the participants were already in-patients, I also talked extensively to them about their experiences prior to admission, expectations once they were referred to the hospice and experiences once admitted. Their responses illustrate significant misunderstandings around the aim or purpose of in-patient hospice or specialist palliative care, although there was significant variation in how this impacted on them emotionally:

> *Participant* (female): Well, I didn't know what the palliative care involved ... you hear all these stories like, "Oh well, that's the end", you know, "once you get into palliative care mate, you've had it," you know, "you're on your last legs". And I said, "No I'm not, I'm not going to do it, I'm not ready yet". And I've made up my mind, I am not ready, and as long as I can hang on, I am going to hang on. [1]

Another respondent comments:

> *Participant* (male): Yeah, I think I might have misunderstood what they were talking about [when discussing palliative care] ... I thought they would have helped me along the road to the suicide, and I don't think that was their criteria at any time ... But [the doctor] still gave me the impression that they would've helped me, with either a morphine needle straight through, or some similar type of drug to ... It was my mistake on that. I do accept the fact that they did not, um, they weren't into this sort of business. I don't really understand what you mean by palliative care, when you, you don't do anything substantial and so forth, you don't help people along.

Another respondent comments:

> *Participant* (female): I wasn't sure what would happen ... No it didn't, no look [the idea of the hospice] really didn't bother me, as far as I'm concerned, palliative care is just another form of caring, by somebody who's in a slightly different field. I know I'm going to die. I mean, it's not a nice thought really, but it happens to all of us.

As shown in the above excerpts, there were diverse understandings and expectations of in-patient hospice care and also levels of fear or hope associated with these understandings. There was a consistent sense of disjunction between expectation and reality, with the focus tending to be on the lack of help in dying (or what some term active euthanasia) and the misnomer that entering the hospice in-patient unit was 'the end'. The former was a huge disappointment for several interviewees and a source of outright frustration, whereas the latter, produced heightened fear in relation to entering the hospice. Paradoxically, the hospice was viewed as more relaxed and positive than anticipated, but also lacking the potency to 'finish things off' due to a combination of politics, legalities and a perceived palliative care culture of 'letting things be' (see also Kelly et al. 2002). This inescapable tension was articulated frequently by the interviewees. These expectations

---

1 Details of participants' specific conditions and ages have in many cases been removed to retain anonymity.

and understandings were critical in the transition to the hospice in-patient unit; a key and emotional moment for each of the participants.

### *Transitions to, and Experiences of, the Hospice*

Previous research, and the data I presented in the previous chapter, indicates that transitional issues (from oncology–palliation; palliation–palliative care) can be particularly difficult for patients and their carers (Schulman-Green et al. 2004). In many cases, fears around the meanings and implications of these transitions can result in a person not actually receiving in-patient hospice care and remaining at home (Hayley et al. 2001). While in many cases staying at home may be appropriate, there also exists the possibility that the *transition* to and myths surrounding in-patient hospice care is the difficulty, rather than the hospice in-patient facility itself. I wanted to explore this transition from the perspective of some of those who had made it. As indicated in the following excerpts, their experiences were varied in relation to transitional phases, with each interviewee experiencing uncertainty, fear and stigma on entering the 'in-patient hospice phase', but also a sense of relief:

> *Participant* (male): Well the day the doctor said I should come in here, I didn't know what to expect, I just didn't know, I thought, "Oh, is this the end? Or what's this going to be?" But within an hour of getting here I could see, you know, that it was just a cancer-type hospital and everyone was, you know, they didn't just bring me here to die, they were bringing me here to help me, type of thing. Oh, I was dubious [before coming], very dubious, I didn't know what. Now I know, I've even told my family about palliative care, if I die, I hope it's here.

Another respondent comments:

> *Participant* (female): Oh [coming to the hospice] was terrible! I came from the [hospital] ... so all I heard was that, "when you come here you die." And that's what scared me. The hospital nurses … one of them said, "You're going to the hospice?" and I said, "Yes," and she said, "I won't see you again then." … she said, "People that go there die." And that shocked me, scared me … I was petrified. I was in pain, I was really sick … [then] my friend told me about the hospice, and she said, "No, you're wrong, it's this, this and this," which is what it is. Um, it's a good place to be, um, it's the best thing I've done …

Another respondent comments:

> *Interviewer*: What was coming to the hospice like, if you don't mind me asking?

> *Participant* (female): Very daunting, very scary ... um, yeah quite – quite scary … I think people need to know more, uh, more of ... people need to be aware of what's going on … So I think more media, media advertising and that, because people are very, uh ... they aren't involved in it at all, uh ...

Another respondent comments:

> *Participant* (male): I've had no quarrel with it. I've had no problems whatsoever, they've been nothing but kind and courteous. It's been really, it's been good, because I really did fight it for a while, coming in. But that's, I think when you get to my stage, you'll find that with a lot of people, you sort of fight coming into a hospice, because you know it's end stage and you just get that feeling sometimes, "Well, if I go in, I might not come home."

There was a real sense of trepidation in the transition to in-patient hospice care, but also a sense of relief for some participants once the comforts of it were revealed. As shown in the excerpts and in other conversations during the interviews, off-the-cuff remarks regarding the hospice in-patient facility by hospital staff often heightened the difficulties of the transition. This was combined with an overwhelming sense that there was a lack of community awareness regarding the roles and meanings of in-patient hospice care. Throughout the interviews significant discontent regarding myth and forms of cultural hearsay regarding in-patient hospice care became apparent.

Within the discussions in and around transitions, 'home' and what home means emerged as a critical issue, drawing emotional and often conflicting responses from the participants. Specifically, 'home' was concurrently desired and feared; it was seen as a place of potential loss of control that could result in a burden for carers, and it could be frightening for the individual (see also McPherson, Wilson and Murray 2007). The hospice in-patient facility, on the other hand, was viewed as enabling the regaining of a *form* of control, albeit an externalised and structurally-determined form. Yet, and as I examine in more detail below, home was inextricably tied to the maintenance of self and identity, resulting in tensions between the need for 'control' and the need to retain a sense of self.

While several of those interviewed found the hospice a more positive and comforting place than anticipated, this was not consistent throughout all the interviews. Several patients experienced a disjunction between need and support, with problematic forms of staff–patient communication perceived as heightening this problem. Particularly in the context of patients who had experienced a swift transition or deterioration, the hospice in-patient facility presented a perilous space of helplessness and even hopelessness. Often desperate to 'get better' and throw themselves into 'any treatment', there was persistent anger expressed throughout these interviews:

> *Participant* (male): I thought the point of being over here [at the hospice] was to teach me how to get mobile again. I mean I'm paralysed from the waist down. I thought the idea was to teach me how to use my body, to get in and out of bed and that, with help. I know I will never, I won't say never, but it will be a long time before I can use my legs, but I thought that was the whole idea. But they [physiotherapists] have only been over twice, so you know, I'm a little disappointed in that … It's just different to what I thought it would be, that's all … I don't really know what they had planned for me. Maybe I'm wrong about thinking that … maybe they think I'm not ready to be taught. I don't know … it is as though I've been forgotten about …

The tensions between 'rehabilitation' and 'treatment' in a context of terminal illness were clear in several of the interviews. Several participants would emphasise the importance to them of the staff not giving up, helping them get better and working towards 'going home'. Often in such cases, staff were (silently) anticipating quick deterioration that was perceived to make a major intervention or rehabilitation 'pointless'. Informal comments were often made by staff before and after the interviews of the dire state of a particular interviewee and their 'unrealistic' expectations. In turn, the need to maintain a positive and hopeful environment in many ways feeds into this predicament.

### *Fun, Play and the Hospice as a Space for Living*

While forms of physical and emotional suffering were dominant themes in the interviews, so too was the notion of the hospice in-patient unit as about living not just dying. Humour was talked about as common in the hospice and represents an under-studied but very important part of end-of-life care (Adamle and Ludwick 2005). A significant number of the interviewees held great importance in the feeling that they were still 'alive' and 'having fun'. With good humour, the hospice in-patient unit and its staff were seen to create an environment where they could maintain a sense of 'living life', in a context of 'doing death':

> *Participant* (male): I'm going out for dinner tonight, I've got some really smart looking clothes to wear, and I'm doing it. Let's go, absolutely. I don't feel like [I'm dying] at all, not even a little bit. I don't feel in any way constrained about what I want to do and how I want to do it. I mean, I get tired, but that's okay, I'll come back and get into bed when I get tired it's not hard to fix. And here [the hospice], I think this place is fantastic, quite frankly, and it's a great place to be, um, the people are just great.

Another respondent comments:

> *Participant* (male): I am very happy, very happy indeed, yes, I am very happy. It's ah, and they treat you as somebody, and they'll even, if they come here and you're sitting on the toilet, they'll stand at the door and bloody have a yak to you. I mean, that's great …

Another respondent comments:

> *Participant* (female): Yes. I had no idea that it was, um, I don't know the right word, like laid-back. Like I got a shock to see, like, little dogs running around, and this type of thing, you know?

Another respondent comments:

> *Participant* (female): I'm happy, I mean, somebody close to me the other day said, my son, actually said, "How do you feel about all of this?" And I said, "Well, it's going to sound like a strange thing to say but I'm not an unhappy cancer patient". I'm very optimistic about life and stuff. I know I'm dying, if I could just die quietly and peacefully and slowly and steadily, and that would be ok … it's hard for me to say to you that I can spell it out for you any more clearly, I just like it!

For most of the participants it was quite a surprise that the hospice environment could be positive, and more importantly, that they could be positive and happy in the hospice environment. The cultural stigma of it as a place of pain and suffering was viewed as a myth, with the interviewees emphasising the 'normal' things that went on, including chats, cups of tea, an afternoon bar service and laughter. Yet, underplaying such narratives of the hospice as a place for humour and play (which indeed, it was and is), was a sense of what Glaser and Strauss (1968) call 'mutual pretence'. Each person (clinician, patient, carer, volunteer) understands the significance of being in a hospice in-patient facility but pretends that the other does not. There is a potential for disconnection between the biological and the social status of the dying patient (Riley 1983). As shown in the following section, the need to create an atmosphere of grace, resolution and fun, may also be prescriptive in the way patients seek to be accepted and cared for.

### *The Accomplished Death and Loved Patients: The Normativity of Hospice*

A key theme in many of the interviews was the humour and good-natured interactions that took place between staff and patients, and between the patients themselves. Yet, there was also an interesting process underlying these relationships: the performative nature of being a 'good' patient and an emphasis on what has been called 'the accomplished death'. This relates to Li's (2004) notion of 'symbiotic niceness' in palliative care more broadly. Specifically, there was a sense that, in order to create a positive hopeful environment, there was a need to be entertaining, cheerful and a 'loved patient'. It was not that one would be abandoned or treated badly by the staff if this was not done, but rather the importance of *being loved* in making the hospice a 'good space' to be and die in:

> *Participant* (female): I like it here … and, um, mind you it helps that I'm also great. They [the staff] like being with me, cause I'm fun to be around, so they enjoy my company as much as I enjoy theirs and yeah it's good, it's an interactive balancing act and we seem to get it together pretty well.

Another respondent comments:

> *Participant* (female): I feel very respected, I'm treated with respect, the nurses treat me with respect. I have lots of fun, they make me laugh, I make them laugh.

Another respondent comments:

> *Interviewer*: It sounds like the staff are enjoying it too.
>
> *Participant*: I've got to [be happy], I've got to, if I don't, imagine if I didn't.
>
> *Interviewer*: What's left?
>
> *Participant*: What have I got? I lost my husband two years ago, he had a heart attack and died. I've got a son with cancer. You know? I haven't got a lot …. Um, because they keep me going, make me laugh.
>
> *Interviewer*: And, you make them laugh.
>
> *Participant* (female): Yeah, exactly. Exactly [exclamation].

It is important to emphasise that I am not arguing that 'the accomplished death' or the performative aspects of patient-clinician interaction are necessarily negative. In many ways the excerpts above were positive reflections on important interpersonal interactions. However, it is important to reflect on what types of talk and expressions meet with 'success', and which demeanours and roles are less well received. While being a 'loved patient' is clearly not problematic per se, one's ability to *be loved* or present a lovable persona are also clearly important factors. There exists a moral dimension to such processes as also discussed by Li and Arber (2006). There can emerge a negotiated order, whereby patients are characterised and even posited as 'troubled' or 'loved' patients. While rapport and intimacy will inevitably be differential in interpersonal relationships within the hospice, patient idiosyncrasies (physical, cultural and psychological) will interplay with, facilitate *and* delimit 'being loved' and the performativity accomplished death.

## *Nostalgia and the Home–Hospice Dialectic*

The tension between being home versus being in a hospice at end of life was a central theme in the interviewees' accounts (see also Thomas, Morris and Clark 2004). The majority of the participants reflected on the importance of and their nostalgia for home, but they also emphasised the importance of the hospice in gaining some control of the end of life. In particular, 'home' seemed central to maintaining a sense of self and identity, which was in turn seen to be (in part) lost in the hospice in-patient unit. The home–hospice tension was ubiquitous in the interviews, often culminating in nostalgic referencing to an 'old self' but also a fear of loss of control and the burden of home:

> *Participant* (male): You know I, I won't say that I'd be disappointed or anything, but if I had a preference, I would prefer not to be back in here within the next month, sort of thing, yeah. You know, I'd like to have some time, at home, as useless as I am.
>
> *Interviewer*: No-one's useless though.
>
> *Participant*: Oh well, I am compared to what I used to be able to do and that, that is the thing that sort of annoys and narks, and I suppose it annoys and narks everyone who's in this position. That you can't get out and do things like mowing lawns, simple bloody things, that you used to be able to do before .... I mean, when we're at home, we [him and his wife] may go half the day without even talking to each other, I'll be sitting in my chair reading a book, she'll be sitting in her chair reading a book, but at the same time, we have that rapport.

Another respondent comments:

> *Participant* (female): But at home, I mean, I've got a much nicer outlook than I do here, and, um, it's just, yeah more comfort, and I just, I feel better at home, I guess ...

Another participant comments:

> *Participant* (male): Now with me not being there, it has given her [his wife] that opportunity. Ah, I know that immediately if I go home, it's going to be the same thing again, I will be number one and she will push herself into the background … She, at the end of the day, she must look forward to her future, not mine, it's hers. She has a right to another couple of years …

Permeating the interviews was nostalgia for home and the 'old self' that home represented. Often this was posited as the 'productive' and 'independent' self that was not a burden on family and partners (see McPherson, Wilson and Murray 2007). Most of the participants felt an ongoing tension between the desire to return home and the perceived safety of the hospice in-patient unit. Perceived loss of self in the hospice was balanced with a sense of the need to reduce the burden on carers and find a method of control over their disintegrating body. Both decisions potentially produced a sense of loss of self; one creating a sense of foreign and unacceptable reliance on others (home) and the other being a foreign environment that created a sense of dislocation from the old self (as the husband, the wife, the gardener and so on). Accepting hospice in-patient care was a strategy to alleviate the burden on others and to reduce the negative impact on themselves (McPherson, Wilson and Murray 2007). However, entering the hospice in turn created a sense of dislocation and a sensory change whereby time–space realities shifted, intermingling with a sense of loss of the 'old self' and further complicating, for some, the preservation of identity.

### *Liminality and Loss of Self in the Hospice*

Within the interviews, a key theme to emerge was the character and feelings associated with the hospice in-patient environment as a quasi-hospital that was comforting but *also* enhanced a sense of disintegration. Specifically, the hospice atmosphere and being in the hospice was talked about as a kind of liminal state or space (Navona and Morag 2004) – that is, one bereft of the recognised parts of one's self, home and identity:

> *Interviewer*: Being in this environment, how does it feel?
>
> *Participant* (female): Hard, sometimes. My [pause] how can I put it, it's hard because it is a hospital, it is a place where you've got to come to get better, or whatever, um, but I, I don't know, my integrity has been lost a lot, a heck of a lot … in a lot of ways that I don't feel happy about … I feel sometimes that, I have no self-esteem left, because I'm in a hospital. I think it could be more, um … yeah, I think it could be more, less hospitalised, like a lounge chair, or painted,

> nice colours and, I think that, I think that would help a lot. Yeah, I think you do, you lose yourself. As a person, as an individual, I think you do.

Another respondent comments:

> *Interviewer*: Do you want to go home, or are you happy here?
>
> *Participant* (male): Well, it's not a case of being … I'm happy enough here I suppose, but every day is the same … I wake up at about five o'clock, half past four, that's after about two hours sleep of course, and you press the button and there's nobody there.

Another respondent comments:

> *Participant* (female): I guess what I expected from the hospice [in-patient unit] was pretty much what there is. Like, I knew it would be a hospital, regardless of how it was decked out. It's still a hospital after all, but with a little more freedom.

Several participants talked about a sense of being in a suspended state, lacking a sense of time and space, and feeling a sense of dislocation from the self (or integrity). The interviewees often discussed the biographical disruptions and even disintegration of being at end-of-life and some may argue that this is an inevitable element of the dying experience, regardless of being in the hospice in-patient unit. Indeed, Little et al. (1998) highlight the potential for liminal states throughout a cancer patient's illness journal. However, in the hospice in-patient unit this seems enhanced given the physical, emotional and spiritual disruptions faced by many patients. The sense of marginality and social disruption of the self pervades this environment, and seems to be facilitated by the increasing institutional and medicalised character of end-of-life care (James and Field 1992). For several participants, in everyday hospice life there was a sense of chat but not conversation; an institutional framework that was cheerful, but not truly engaging. Again, reminiscent of Li's (2004) 'symbiotic niceness', several felt like the rush of the institution and the limited conversations with staff were alienating and caused a sense of dislocation and isolation:

> *Participant* (female): I know I've got to have a certain amount of rest in bed, but basically you'd think that in a building this size, there would always be someone to talk to. There isn't! Yes, I thought, "This is going to be so different, I'll have all these new people to communicate with". But it's not like that at all. The nurses are so busy, they haven't got time for chit-chat. Um, and even the person in the bed next to me … I mean I say what I can to her, but, um, she's down in the dumps.

As shown in the above excerpt and in several of the other interviews, there was a sense that interpersonal interactions may be performative or perhaps fleeting (and for a reason). As one participant commented, 'I felt she was listening, but she didn't want to stay long, she was really wanting to go'. In contrast to the accounts presented earlier which emphasised the hospice as a site for play, chat and fun, several participants struggled with the coping strategies of staff members seeking to balance empathy and kindness with workloads and the potential distress of working with people who are dying. The resulting interactional dynamic contributed to the sense of dislocation and disruption in the social self and the integrity of everyday interactions. There is clearly a dissociative element to palliative care work which Fox (2006) labels as 'detached concern'. Several participants commented on the importance for the hospice environment of 'not taking things too seriously' and 'maintaining a positive environment'. In other studies caregivers also described their communication with patients about the end of life as being subtle or indirect with no tacit acknowledgment of the patient's prognosis (see Schulman-Green et al. 2004). As such, I do not suggest that this approach is inherently flawed; however, it does feed into the impacts and even limitations of hospice in-patient care.

## Discussion

In this chapter I have sought to interrogate some of the contemporary issues around particular forms of institutional dying, with an emphasis on experiences in the last few weeks of life in an in-patient hospice unit. This is set within a broader context where the majority of people are not dying at home, and there is a significant expansion of in-patient specialist palliative care and hospice services in Australia and many other OECD countries. I embarked on this analysis to explore how shifts in available places for dying may be inflecting the experience of dying. The broader desire was to develop a critical sociology of this (relatively) new space for dying.

A key theme emergent from the interviews was the disjunctions between expectations, understandings and the actual hospice experience (see also Hayley et al. 2001). This disjunction operated on two levels: surprising positivity (not the space of death and dying as expected), and frustration (an inability to assist in death). The misnomers and cultural myths in and around hospice care were central to such disjunctions and often the trauma of entry was the most difficult element in what was otherwise experienced as a (relatively) positive experience. Furthermore, the perceived legal and medical agendas, versus those of death with dignity (in all its permutations) were viewed as problematic when assumptions about what could be done were reconciled with the realities of in-patient hospice care.

In trying to understand and conceptualise the decisions regarding in-patient hospice care, I focused on the values underpinning key decisions including whether to stay at home or enter the in-patient unit. A sense of 'control', or lack thereof, was a central theme in the participants' decisions to enter in-patient hospice care, in that home was concurrently viewed and experienced as a site of comfort and of fear. The hospice in-patient unit represented a means of taking control (reducing reliance on family) while also of losing control (submitting to the institutionalised medical regime). This home–help dialectic centred on the need to balance a desire and longing for a sense of home and self (Exley and Letherby 2001), while not sacrificing one's family or partner's life. The notion of 'burden' was central to such discourses, positioning the institution as a means of ameliorating the pain and loss of livelihood perceived to occur when families have to cope with a person dying at home. Identity disruption and disintegration permeated these discussions, with the need to balance an impossible combination of needs, that is, loss of self associated with being a burden, versus loss of self in opting for an environment away from one's home, community and sense of identity. A complex dialectical tension emerged between nostalgia for home (and the old self) and nostophobia, the fear of coming home.

The environment of the hospice in-patient unit also held a plethora of contradictions, presenting a space of hope and life, but also of complex emotions and struggles around authenticity and identity. There emerged a sense of liminality central to the in-patient hospice experience (Froggatt 1997; Navona and Morag 2004), marked by various degrees of disorientation, sense of inter-personal inauthenticity, loss of self and transitionality. Such feelings of liminality seem closely tied to the cultures of practice amongst hospice in-patient staff, many of whom focus on hope and cheer as a way of coping and creating a positive environment for patients, carers and fellow clinicians. For some patients, this may promote a sense of dislocation from the reality of their situation, and disrupt a sense of authenticity within interpersonal dynamics (Fox 2006). Moreover, the types of spaces and places within the hospice seem to give fewer temporal, cultural, and personal cues and signifiers that engender a sense of life and vitality (see also Froggatt 1997). I do not argue that this is either necessarily avoidable or problematic for *all* patients. The appeal of in-patient hospice care, for some, lies in its potential to create an environment without the trauma of potential uncontrolled pain and distress; to help ease the transition between life and death without the 'burden' on family and friends. Yet, the spaces it creates and the forms of interactionality it promotes may also result in very specific forms of social and identity disintegration.

The appeal of the hospice is, I argue, the flip-side of its limitations. Providing a manageable space whereby some degree of control maybe regained (and the burden on family reduced) creates a semi-liminal space, less interactionally authentic than that of home (at least when nostalgically framed), prioritising the physical management of symptoms (James and Field 1992; McNamara 2004). However, the creation of an environment focused on promoting cheer and life, in turn, opens up the potential for the performativity of a good death; death as something that can be accomplished so as to be cared for and viewed by staff in the best way possible (Hart, Sainsbury and Short 1998). Also observed in studies of nurses' talk in the hospice in-patient unit (patients as 'very difficult' or 'a darling') we see the ways in which the hospice experience is fundamentally shaped by patients interactions with and demands that they make on hospice staff (Li and Arber 2006).

Linking back to the need for authenticity and a sense of recognition, the pressures to be 'accomplished in death' may be very strong for many people in the hospice in-patient unit. Such ideas and discursive devices are socially endorsed and embedded (Sontag 1991) and, I argue, perhaps fundamentally problematise authenticity in interpersonal contact. Symbiotic niceness (Li 2004), and the need to be and perform competency when dying, may undermine the authenticity of interactions, and create a greater or more drawn out sense of the social death or disintegration of self (Glaser and Strauss 1968; Lawton 1998; Rozmovits and Ziebland 2004; Sacks and Nelson 2007). As a patient once reflected after an interview, 'I've done a lot of dying already'.

Clearly, further exploration is needed to examine a wider range of experiences in different in-patient contexts. Yet, what these interviews do reveal is some of the interpersonal, structural and medico-cultural processes shaping contemporary experiences near death. This area would benefit significantly from further sociological work focused on conceptualising contemporary in-patient hospice experiences, including the accounts of other stakeholders including carers and volunteers. The following chapter continues with the hospice theme, exploring in detail the ethical and moral conundrums presented by this environment, focusing on patient/participant perspectives on how questions around assisted dying and religiosity are played out within the hospice. That is, how the hospice morally bounds patients, asking of them certain things, and disallowing certain deaths.

# Chapter 4
# The Moralities and Politics of Dying in a Hospice

> … one of the guys [here at the hospice] was saying to me, "People say dying is like walking through the gates of hell". He says, "Well, I believe we are walking through the gates of hell, but we're walking out of hell". (Hospice in-patient, Male)

## Introduction

Dying is a decidedly moral event. In many respects, it is a series of moral performances by an individual, their family and carers. It is also a morally-regulated event whereby certain experiences are allowed and fostered and others are denied. What we do and feel in the context of dying is heavily shaped by sociocultural expectations and pressures regarding *how to die*. Sociologically speaking, dying is thus a morally-laden site of illness and care, bound by evolving and often institutionally-governed cultural and social norms (Broom and Cavenagh 2010, 2011). Dying involves negotiating and often resisting important and at times problematic social dynamics of gift, reciprocity and obligation (Chattoo and Ahmad 2008; Frank 1997). It is shaped by a moral economy of illness and care that provides a culturally-specific and relational framework for 'dying well' (Booth 1994). 'Living up to' these cultural scripts around dying is an important social dynamic for individuals who are dying and for their carers and families (Kellehear 2008). In this chapter I focus on unpacking the presence of specific normative expectations around dying – what I call the moral fabric of dying – as this is played out within a hospice.

Within the modern moral economy of dying, two high profile and contested issues are those of *assisted dying* and the role of *religiosity* within formal care settings (Eliott and Olver 2008). They represent perhaps the extremes of the moral–immoral cultural binary of 'dying well' (Gott et al. 2008). Religious guidance is viewed by many as central to a morally 'good ending' – dying as a natural or spiritual transition involving practices of 'redemption' and 'finding peace'. Assisted dying is viewed by many as a culturally 'immoral practice' involving an 'unnatural' ending or even a 'cop-out' in an otherwise natural process. Thus both assisted dying and religiosity are part of the broader moral construction of dying.

While assisted dying and religious input may be informally negotiated when an individual dies at home, when an individual dies in an institutional setting the institution (in many respects) governs the moral and ethical underpinnings of dying (Payne, Langley-Evans and Hillier 1996; see also Seale 1998b). As also outlined in Chapter 3, the institutionalising of dying offers new opportunities but it also *governs* dying, sometimes shaping *when* a person is able to die (timing and assisted dying) and shaping the *meaning* of dying (providing religious guidance and existential advice). Given this, significant questions remain unanswered including: How hospices manage ethical questions around justice, self-determination, individual agency in the timing and character of death? and How hospices honour spiritual and religious beliefs without reifying religion as a necessary part of 'dying well'?

As outlined in the previous chapters, the modern hospice as an institution attempts to meet a range of patient needs, including those related to physical, emotional and spiritual wellbeing. In doing so, hospice and specialist in-patient palliative care necessarily blur the line between formalised medical expertise and cultural or religious belief systems. As opposed to other areas of medicine that are largely disease focused, palliative and end-of-life care are intimately involved in the management of emotions and existential issues within their patient population. This highly diversified site of healthcare delivery has evolved to contain subtle political positionings and embedded cultural values that are often concealed in other biomedical contexts (Edmondson et al. 2008; see also Exline and Yali 2000). Once in institutions, patients and their families are exposed to a range of frameworks which may either allow or limit certain things, including an accelerated death (James and Field 1992; Johansen et al. 2005).

In this chapter I explore just some of the ethics and moralities of dying within the hospice setting, focusing on questions of assisted dying and the role of religiosity. This involves unpacking how hospices may allow *and* disallow certain things at the end of life and how hospices can problematise a sense of human agency and self-determination. I draw on previous work on moral economies (cf. Booth 1994; Chattoo and Ahmad 2008) to explore how such institutions produce and govern ideas about 'good' and 'timely' deaths and, in turn, frame experiences of dying. Before exploring the experiences of Australian hospice patients themselves, I explore some of the scholarly work in the area.

## Background

### *The Right to Die and the Institutional Mediation of Dying*

Euthanasia/assisted dying and religiosity are controversial and politically-laden issues within the broader community, and within the hospice the emotions surrounding them are even more acute. They are inseparable issues given that existential questions have driven much of the lobbying against euthanasia and assisted dying (that is, not 'playing God'). Debate has been ongoing in the popular press, in the community and in the academic and medical literature (Givens and Mitchell 2009), with high levels of disagreement over its place in modern medicine (Emanuel et al. 1996) or its validity from a human rights perspective (Dowbiggin 2002). Hitherto, most academic literature in relation to euthanasia and assisted dying has sought to examine the issues in terms of: the possibility of consent; the capacity to choose; changes in views over time; the moralities of care; and medico-legal risk (e.g. Eliott and Olver 2007; Mak et al. 2005; Mohammed and Peter 2009). Few studies have qualitatively explored terminal patients' views about euthanasia, assisted dying and religiosity (Eliott and Olver 2008; Nissim, Gagliese and Rodin 2009; Somerville 2003) despite recognition of the need to document patient perspectives (Mak, Elwyn and Finlay 2003; Mak and Elwyn 2005) and research with clinicians that illustrate the intensity and importance of such issues in patient care (Denier et al. 2010). This is a gap I begin to fill in this chapter.

There has been considerable research on end-of-life preferences among different groups of patients (e.g. Breitbart et al. 2000; Emanuel et al. 1996; Johansen et al. 2005; Kelly et al. 2002; Kuuppelomäki 2000; Parkinson et al. 2005), although mostly in community or out-patient settings. There also is a significant body of social science literature on euthanasia, desire for hastened death and assisted suicide (e.g. Donchin 2000; Givens and Mitchell 2009; McPherson, Wilson and Murray 2007; Seale and Addington-Hall 1994). A significant proportion of this work has focused on the views of cancer patients who are dying and their perspectives on euthanasia (e.g. Eliott and Olver 2007, 2008) or desire for a hastened death (e.g. Breitbart et al. 2000). The majority of this work has also been informed by psychosocial or biomedical perspectives, particularly on the role of depression, grief and 'hopelessness' as predictors of a desire for hastened death (Breitbart et al. 2000). Such work, while important for emphasising supportive care needs at the end of life, can risk reconstructing and representing individual patient preferences for a hastened death or assisted dying as environmental or as about 'better case management' rather than an authentic individual desire for a quicker death. For example, in their research Johansen et al. (2005) state that the wish to die is an ambivalent and fluctuating mental 'solution' for the future arguing that health care providers should be aware of this when responding to utterances regarding euthanasia. Such assumptions about the psychological underpinnings of euthanasia requests permeate hospice care, as evident in the results presented here.

## *Autonomy and Moralities*

While I acknowledge that in some cases desire for a hastened death may stem from resolvable psychological issues or gaps in supportive care, it remains a possibility that for others it is a legitimate desire that persists over time. The debates raise complex issues about individual autonomy and the right of 'rational competent adults' to make decisions regarding ending their life voluntarily (Donchin 2000; see also Dowbiggin 2002). The possibility of a person as autonomous decision maker or whether autonomy is ultimately relationally produced and enacted remains a debated issue (Donchin 2000). In the context of the hospice – to an even greater extent than in other health contexts – carers, family members and clinicians all influence and shape the patient's wants, fears and hopes (Kellehear 2008), which further problematises ideas about individual autonomy and agency (Frank 1997). This speaks to the intersubjective character of dying I outlined in the Introduction. Moreover, discourses around assisted dying and religiosity reflect the broader moral economy of living and dying in a hospice (Broom and Cavenagh 2010, 2011; Chattoo and Ahmad 2008; Sivaramakrishnan 2005; Booth 1994). The saliency of issues surrounding death and dying constitutes the hospice as a key site of moral practice; an inter-subjective process involving the production and reconstitution of the 'competent social agent' takes place (Chattoo and Ahmad 2008). Moral practice, in this context, denotes ideas about how people should treat others and be treated by them, including, as Sayer (2005) posits, matters of justice and fairness, and relations of recognition, care and friendship. Such moral codes also produce interpersonal and cultural dynamics around responsibility, gift and reciprocity (Frank 1997) which in turn shape the dying process (Broom and Cavenagh 2010, 2011).

The moral underpinnings of cancer and cancer care have been emphasised previously by other authors. As Seale (2001) has argued, the discursive and rhetorical practices often utilised by palliative and hospice care clinicians, carers and other stakeholders ('be strong' or 'fight hard'), morally bind patient choice and desire, producing 'good patients' as well as 'good deaths' (Broom and Cavenagh 2010, 2011; Broom and Tovey 2008). Likewise, contemporary Australian hospice care is still largely informed by particular models of 'dying well'. The 'revivalist' good death, for example, has been an agenda within palliative care that espouses being pain free, acceptance, closure, awareness and individuality among other things (Clark 2002: 907; Seale 1998). While such components are not prima facie problematic, their normative and prescriptive potential is worth considering. These models of 'dying well' have tended to be driven by academic and clinical perspectives, with little research evidence available on how these ideas resonate with patients' views (Gott et al. 2008). Such moral codes around 'dying well' intermingle with the politics of assisted dying and the role of religiosity in the hospice.

### *Euthanasia/Assisted Dying and the Hospice*

Within the in-patient hospice or specialist palliative care context, wider philosophical debates about rights versus ethics or psychosocial status versus autonomy are often implicit and unspoken. Within an institution, in the last few weeks of life patient desire for 'an end' versus 'fighting on' can be difficult to express given the audience and stakeholders listening to such 'talk' (see Breitbart et al. 2000; Donchin 2000). The hospice, as an institution, offers a specific model of managing dying (Clark 2002; James and Field 1992): in theory at least, a dying process with as little pain as possible and with various supportive mechanisms to assist in a 'comfortable death' (Kubler-Ross 1969). Yet, what is perceived by patients as the role of the hospice and what is actually experienced within the hospice may be considerably different. Indeed, euthanasia and assisted suicide operates largely outside the hospice setting (within the community). When entering the hospice, a person is exposed to certain ideological views on dying and institutional practices of 'maintaining' life (till a 'natural death') that are often unexpected, and for some, even unwanted. Euthanasia or assisted dying is not considered a part of Australian hospice care and, as shown in other studies of palliative care contexts, staff are often reticent about interventions that are perceived to accelerate death (Rietjens et al. 2007). This brings to the fore the degree to which hospice care is implicated in and inflecting people's dying processes, particularly for those who seek or even expect an accelerated death. The hospice, I argue here, represents a site of contemporary governance of the 'timely death' (Parry 1982, 1994); a manifestation of a broader set of social contracts of rights (such as, the right to dignity, life and so on) that the modern nation state is obliged to provide. As we see in the following sections, such rights come with responsibilities allowing certain possibilities and limiting human agency. Furthermore, such hospice values have tended to emerge, at least in part, from Christian religious values and this history still underpins and informs contemporary hospice care.

### *Religiosity in the Hospice*

As I suggested in the Introduction, many hospices in Australia have emerged from, and continue to espouse, certain religious notions of acceptance, faith and redemption. The Christian underpinnings of elements of hospice care continue to shape people's experiences of end-of-life care and, ultimately, much hospice care represents an intimate interplay of medicalisation and religiosity (Ardelt and Koenig 2006). Although biomedical and nursing technologies and expertise remain at the fore of explicit reasons for entering the hospice, the day-to-day realities of in-patient hospice care involve a multifaceted environment that contains religious undertones of, and sometimes explicit reference to, resolution and acceptance. While patients are not asked or pushed to 'talk religion', nor is religion pushed on them, the types of services offered (that is, a Christian chaplain and a chapel) provide a certain framing of dying that is situated within a Catholic tradition in the case of the hospice examined in this chapter.

Catholicism has been stridently against euthanasia or assisted dying, perceiving 'suicide' as an unforgivable sin. This has been reflected in regular statements and lobbying from the Vatican. On 2 February 2009, Pope Benedict XVI stated that euthanasia was a false solution to the drama of suffering (Baklinski 2009). While religion is fundamental to the dying experience for many people (see Sulmasy 2006), there are debates around religion-as-coping (see Exline and Yali 2000; Pargament et al. 2004) and the pressure or guilt associated with the allure of religiosity at the end of life (Exline and Yali 2000). In the hospice context, the moral framing of dying from a religious perspective may become intertwined with formalised models of 'dying well', including Kubler-Ross's stages of dying (see Kubler-Ross 1969). Formalised palliative care models of 'dying well' may interplay, perhaps subtly and differentially depending on the organisation, with religious ideas about 'acceptance', 'moving on' and dying as 'a stage'.

In the following section, drawing on my interviews with people in the last few weeks of life living in an Australian hospice, I focus on how people reflect on, negotiate, and at times resist, the available resources for dying in the hospice, that is, how they perceive and manage the pressures, allure and comforts of particular endings. Religious support within the hospice, I argue, is intimately intertwined with the moral framings of the right to die, constructions of timely deaths, and hospice care belief systems around 'acceptance' and 'resolution'.

## Into the Field

### *Hospice Patients' Perspectives on 'Assisted' Dying and the Right to Die*

As with the previous chapter, here I draw on a series of interviews and a period of ethnographic work involving 20 hospice in-patients in the last few weeks (or days) of their lives in New South Wales, Australia. At the cusp of death, I had the privilege of discussing with them the complex and sensitive issues related to assisting dying and the desire for a hastened death. It is extremely rare to document the perspectives of people within weeks and days of death. The process of asking such questions about assisted dying and religiosity was not without its difficulties in the hospice environment, both in terms of staff perspectives and patient and family sensitivities. The hospice as a collective unit was focused on ideas about 'acceptance' and 'comfort' with no explicit discussion allowed or ideological acceptance of 'accelerating' the dying process. Yet, the issue of an accelerated death, 'helping me along' or explicit euthanasia, kept emerging in my discussions with the participants and largely without prompting. The hospice management would talk about such thought processes in their patients as representing a need for 'more counsel' or 'more support from staff and carers'. Talk of euthanasia and 'ending it' was viewed in my informal conversations with staff as a 'cry for help'. While it is not my aim here to resolve this tension, the hospice staff's broad dismissal of patients' desires for accelerated death creates a range of moral and ethical tensions that were important to the participants. As we see below, staff and patients both had strong feelings about rights and dying, many of which had been enhanced by a disjunction between their expectations and the realities of hospice care:

> *Participant*: I think they should have the same system as what the Dutch have, self-euthanasia, I believe in that, I think it should be like, you press a button and you say goodbye.
>
> *Interviewer*: The right to die?
>
> *Participant*: The right to die. I mean it's no good having people, it's no good shooting seven thousand dogs a year, which is what they do in [specific Australian State], and leaving the humans to suffer, you know, that to me is not right, that's what I think anyway.
>
> *Interviewer*: How do you think the hospice view it?
>
> *Participant* (male): I don't think they think of it. Most of them would just be getting the salary, that's their main worry, feeding their families. It's only when you reach the stage that I'm at, that ah, you start thinking about these things. I'm probably a little bit too severe when I'm talking about dogs, but it's only a manner of speech.

Each of the participants held strong perspectives on the prospect of, or debates around, euthanasia or assisting dying. There was virtually unanimous support for an 'accelerated death' if requested and this was broadly how euthanasia and assisted dying was construed and articulated in the interviews. There was a general view that the hospice was against using technological or pharmaceutical means to accelerate death. This is unsurprising to academic audiences given the philosophy of hospice care and the ideology of 'acceptance' and facilitating 'natural' deaths. However, this *was* surprising to the majority of the participants. The idea of euthanasia or assisted dying was talked about in highly emotive and passionate terms. As shown above, and in many of the other interviews, the idea of a 'natural ending' with closure, acceptance and dignity did not resonate with their experiences. While often communicated in guilt ridden terms ('I suppose I'm being too harsh'), these patients talked about the frustrations of institutionalised dying, the moral frameworks underpinning hospice care and the ethics of prolonging life (or lack thereof). Being treated 'worse than a dog' was a phrase several of the patients used.

One of the interviewee's stories illustrated vividly the potential disjunction between institutionalised models of 'dying well' and individual desire. He had recently attempted to commit suicide at home and, as a result of being 'unsuccessful', had been brought to the hospice. The staff had told the author that he 'needed more support to move beyond his negative outlook' and that it was part of his process:

> *Interviewer*: Well, I always think it's best to start [the interview] where you think it's right to start. Where does it start for you?
>
> *Participant*: When I decided to commit suicide ... [some details removed for confidentiality]. I had had a heart attack ... I was dead in the water ... I couldn't walk and I was weak, and I've always been a fairly strong person, you know, able to do things.
>
> *Interviewer*: So you're losing those core things that you wanted to do?
>
> *Participant*: Yeah, um. They [the hospital out-patient palliative care unit] gave me this morphine derivative [for pain], so I drank it, in one gulp more or less, about 150 mils, and I thought that would help me along. And I think it was working, I don't know, I passed out by this stage. One of my neighbours walked in on me, and she didn't walk away, she rang the bloody ambulance and the doctors, and created a general fuss and here I am.
>
> *Interviewer*: What you said about Palliative Care, and helping you die, 'cause I mean, is that something that you would have liked them to do? Um, to help you in that way?
>
> *Participant*: Oh yeah [exclamation].
>
> *Interviewer*: And why do you think they didn't?
>
> *Participant*: I don't, well they're not allowed to by law to start with, is one of the things. Um, ah, why they didn't do it? Religion would be one, would be the main one I should imagine. And just morality that it's wrong to take a life and so forth. But it's my decision, and I should have been left alone. I do believe this, and I have lots of friends, who my children said that to, "You should have just left him alone. You go, you wanted to go. You've had your life." I'm 83 in nine months.
>
> *Interviewer*: You wanted to go in a painless way?

> *Participant* (male): Yeah, basically … I don't really understand what you mean by palliative care, when you, you don't do anything substantial and so forth, you don't help people along … 'cause you can talk to elderly people, which I do 'cause I'm old and they talk to you, and 95–97 per cent of them agree that we should be able to go when we want to. The law should be changed …

The above excerpt resonates with several of the participants' experiences of managing and at times resisting the hospice model of 'dying well'. While several were extremely focused on living as long as possible (see discussion in this chapter below), this was often situated within a moral framing of 'holding on', 'being strong' and not 'giving up'. There was a clear theme within the participants' accounts of an impotency in the face of hospice 'rules' around intervention (although these were not formalised or explicit). A common reflection was that once you accepted entry into the hospice you were subsumed within its ideological framing of 'the good death'. The majority accepted that this was a reasonable 'sacrifice' in order to lower the burden on family through a more 'controlled' death – again, reminiscent of ideas about gift, reciprocity and obligation (Chattoo and Ahmad 2008; Broom and Cavenagh 2010, 2011). But there was a concurrent sense of entrapment in their accounts. The gift, in this context, is a willingness to embrace or at least accept one's dying process and its permutations. The reciprocity takes the form of a right to die in a more controlled manner, without such a burden being placed on family and carers. Within this moral framework, an accelerated death was not part of the equation and, when verbalised, problematised ideas about reciprocity.

## *Questioning Euthanasia/Assisted Dying and the Desire to Live*

It is important to emphasise that the participants' perspectives on euthanasia or assisted dying were by no means linear and there was significant (albeit minority) support for the hospice being a safe space that was not a 'covert form of euthanasia'. There was an emphasis on living within and enjoying the hospice phase; counter to the participant perspectives examined above, there was support for a clear separation between hospice care and euthanasia or assisted dying. As shown in the second excerpt below, some participants were thriving in an institutionalised dying setting, with no desire (at the point of the interview, anyway) for accelerated death. While more research is needed to explore this, their perspectives came across as not embedded in the specificities of symptomatology (that those in more pain wanted a faster death):

> *Participant* (male): It's ah, it's like the old horse and water situation, you, ah, can open the stable door and you can take the horse out to the pond, but you can't

> make him [sic] drink, sort of thing, you know? So it's up to the individual, too, I think we need to have a lot more awareness of palliative care, what it is … a lot of people are afraid, I think, that, they're sort of getting the feeling that this is sort of "euthanasia by stealth", sort of … it isn't, it's given me a choice …

Another respondent comments:

> *Participant* (male): Well, I didn't know what palliative care involved … you hear all these stories like, "Oh well, that's the end", you know, "once you get into palliative care mate, you've had it," you know, "you're on your last legs". And I said, "No I'm not, I'm not going to do it, I'm not ready yet". And I've made up my mind, I am not ready, and as long as I can hang on, I am going to hang on.

The interviews reinforced the complexities and differentiated perspectives on euthanasia or assisted dying and desire to hasten death, even among a relatively small group of hospice in-patients. Their accounts illustrate the importance of accepting that assisted dying is an important, divisive, contentious and persistent theme within the lived experiences of dying. The hospice staff – at least in this hospice setting – tended to view assisted dying as a subject not appropriate to discuss and a practice that 'doesn't happen in hospice'. Yet, the patients, whether for or against being offered euthanasia/assisted dying, did express a desire for discussion around the issue. As mentioned above, part of the reason that euthanasia and assisted dying is frowned upon in the hospice relates to the Catholic underpinnings of hospice care in Australia. Most of the interviewees talked about religion as the 'unspoken driving force of hospice care'. In the day-to-day running of the project, if a nurse came in during an interview (out of necessity to check on the patient), there would be comments that 'we don't do that here' or 'you're doing alright aren't you, we don't want you to go yet'. These comments and the accounts of the interviewees provide a glimpse into the potential moral underpinnings of a hospice death and the omnipotence of religiosity in hospice care, whether explicit or implicit.

### *Religion, Redemption and the Hospice*

Much like euthanasia, religious beliefs often simmer under the surface of institutionalised end-of-life care settings and day-to-day interactions in hospices, but rarely are they explicitly addressed in clinician–patient interaction. Discussions about afterlives, redemption, god(s) and so on in the hospice seems natural to some extent, but at the same time can be morally laden and culturally bound. And, as discussed in the interviews, the participants experienced such discussions in different ways as difficult, important, divisive and, at times, intolerable. In this study, these issues were brought up naturally and sensitively and none of the interviewees reacted negatively to these discussions. The idea was to examine how they viewed the place of religion as part of formalised hospice care and the role of the chaplain and hospice ideology in their dying process. Each patient had strong opinions on this issue:

> *Interviewer*: Spirituality and religion are obviously, for some people, quite important …
>
> *Participant* (male): Very important.
>
> *Interviewer*: How do you think that's … is that part of what the hospice should be about, is that part of, for you, is that a personal thing, or what?
>
> *Participant*: No, I think it's a personal thing. I mean I don't have any great religion. I do believe that there's something out there. I believe that we go somewhere, I don't believe that we drop off, wherever. I think we've got to go somewhere, the essence of us, has got to go somewhere. But, where that is, I don't know. Call it God, call it karma, call it Santa Claus, who knows! I think it's there, for everybody, I think everybody has their own belief of whatever. But, it should not be part of it [hospice care].

Another respondent comments:

> *Interviewer*: I guess everyone's different, and whether they call it religion or spirituality or whatever, I guess it would be nice if you could tell me about whether you think that has a place in the hospice?
>
> *Participant* (male): No, not in my life it doesn't. None of the above. I'm not religious, nor spiritual … I really do believe that you are born, and that you live, and then you die and in the meantime you do the best you can with what you've got … What happens to me after I die, I don't care. I mean there might be a reward, and I might suddenly go, "Whoa, shit!" But I don't imagine it's going to happen.
>
> *Interviewer*: Do you think that the hospice should be providing sort of, spiritual …
>
> *Participant*: I don't want them to. They asked me that when I came here and I said, "No, I'm fine thanks." So they do, and they will, you know there's a chapel up there if you need to go there, and they have pastoral care, if you care to tell

> them a story about it [your faith], and I just don't, I'm not interested in religion, never have been.

Another respondent comments:

> *Interviewer*: Do you think, for you, is it, is sort of religious and spiritual stuff important for the hospice? Is that important for you?
>
> *Participant* (male): No, no, no, no, no, I don't go on with that sort of thing.
>
> *Interviewer*: Okay. Has the chaplain come along to talk to you at all?
>
> *Participant*: Well they asked me to convert as soon as I come [sic] in the door, and I said, no, I'm not worried about that mate.

Another respondent comments:

> *Participant* (female): No, no. Religion has no business in here. That's for yourself to figure out ...

Evident in the above excerpts, and in the other interviewees' accounts, the role of religion within the hospice and within the institutionalised dying process was controversial and even frowned upon by some participants as inappropriate for a 'medical environment'. Several suggested that religion has 'no business' in a hospice and that whether implicit or explicit they felt pressured to 'think about God' when visited by the chaplain. It should be noted here that in such an emotive environment – and an environment where many people do desire pastoral care – there will always be some who find supportive care ideologically difficult to accept. Yet, there are complexities that deserve further examination, in particular, the hospice as a sphere for conversion, redemption and evangelicalism, and how informal systems operate within a publicly funded medical environment that espouse certain understandings (Christian in this case) of theology, life after death, the meanings of living and dying and so on – that is, the hospice as a grey area between expertise and faith; knowledge and belief; endings and beginnings; and, technologies and ideologies. Before entry, the hospice tends to be viewed as a quasi-hospital environment whereby pain can be controlled and bodily disintegration held in check. However, on admission, the hospice offers, provides and espouses much more than just technologies of pain reduction and symptom control; it offers an ideological model of dying and resources for existential needs much of which, as I illustrate in the following section, are highly valued by patients.

## *Positive Views on Religion in the Hospice*

The interviews revealed significant differentiation in the importance and place of religion in the hospice. The participants were split almost equally in their views on the appropriateness or inappropriateness of Christianity as part of hospice supportive care. Those participants who supported religiosity as part of hospice life were not all explicitly religious (that is, when asked, they did not all claim to be 'Christian'). However, each talked about the comfort and importance of religious guidance and notions of afterlives for their wellbeing within the hospice:

> *Participant* (male): Yes, my wife and I, we have a Christian faith, and we do believe in a life to come, the resurrection and all that. So that sort of, is what I think, buoys us up, and you know, we've got hope for the future.
>
> *Interviewer*: It's not the end?
>
> *Participant*: No, it's not the end.

Another respondent comments:

> *Participant* (female): I often sit in the chapel. I find great comfort from it. I think that that is where a lot of that help comes from. Life's not all about money and all of that, it goes a lot deeper than that … it's not any particular religion or denomination. I prefer to look at it from a spiritual point of view.

Another respondent comments:

> *Interviewer*: In terms of spirituality or religion, however you want to think about it, do you think that is an important part of what the hospice should offer, or is that a personal thing?
>
> *Participant* (male): Well, when you see the hospice and you enter it, it automatically comes to you that it's in a religious place.
>
> *Interviewer*: Right.
>
> *Participant*: … because it, it breathes that kind of thing.
>
> *Interviewer*: It does?

> *Participant*: Which is a very good thing, after all, you couldn't make it a public hospital could you? Everyone running around, clattering here and banging, I mean, it's lovely and peaceful here. So if you want to die anywhere, die in a hospice.
>
> *Interviewer*: And is it something that …
>
> *Participant*: [coughing fit]
>
> *Interviewer*: … is it something that you think should be actively provided? So people coming around and talking about God?
>
> *Participant*: Well I think they have a chaplain, don't they?
>
> *Interviewer*: They do.
>
> *Participant*: Who comes in regularly. I don't think you could get much more than that. The, I think the chaplain should spend a little bit more time, I mean, I haven't seen him around. But I think there should be a chaplain, probably here, maybe two or three hours a day, or maybe two or three hours every two days, I don't know which way they would administer that. I certainly feel that there should be a chaplain ready to talk to people, like, to me.

In many respects these excerpts and those presented above represent the Catch 22 of religious supportive care in the hospice. Religion was talked about in quite diverse ways by the participants and was often talked about as instilling a moral conundrum for their clinicians who were attempting to balance the dying process with cultural resources commonly drawn on to cope with death and loss (such as ideas about an afterlife, eternal life, forgiveness and redemption). My focus here is not on critiquing the presence of religion within the hospice, but rather, on understanding how its presence impacts on patients who enter the space. As I mentioned above, the impacts and experiences of religiosity are actually experienced relationally – like other moral practices and dying rituals – that is, in the hospice, surrounded by other stakeholders, doing 'religion' or not 'doing religion' can have very different meanings and implications.

## *The Pressure to Redeem: Hospice and Carer Expectations*

While not a theme emerging in all the interviews, several patients revealed a pressure from carers and family members for 'acceptance' of their death and 'redemption' through 'God'. They described the broader relational and cultural expectation that one should find a higher meaning or existential closure before dying. At least in part, this was viewed as encouraged by the presence of a hospice chaplain and chapel. The interviews illustrated how in the last few weeks of life some feel pressure from family members and hospice workers to find peace with their impending death. Once again, and this time in the context of religious choices and beliefs, questions about autonomy emerge in an organisational setting involving a complex combination of vulnerability, giving and reciprocity:

> *Participant* (male): A man [sic] has a true belief in God or Buddha, or whoever it may be, and he wants to include that in his death, I think he has the right to state his wishes, and as far as those wishes can be fulfilled, um, I think, between the family and the palliative care service, maybe we should do our best to provide it, because it will make it easier for him [sic] to accept …
>
> *Interviewer*: What about for you?
>
> *Participant*: I'm not a very religious person. I sort of, I don't believe that we human beings are the be-all-and-end-all of this universe, by any means.
>
> *Interviewer*: Do you see that being a personal thing, or something that the Palliative, the Hospice should be involved in?
>
> *Participant*: Well, I believe there's moves to put in that, I've had a guy [chaplain] down here, last Friday and the Friday before, sort of thing, he used to sit here for a few hours, he kind of works non-denominational, he's …
>
> *Interviewer*: You can talk with him?
>
> *Participant*: Yeah.
>
> *Interviewer*: Did you find that useful?
>
> *Participant*: … you know his [the patient's] family might be, he might have one or two saying, "Oh, we need this, we need that," whereas the guy himself might, not need it much, you know.

As illustrated above, and in other interviewee's accounts, acceptance of religious supportive care in the hospice may be, at least in part and for some patients, relational in character: related to carer, family and clinician-driven desire for acceptance and resolution. In this way, the participants articulated a relational ontology of religiosity in the context of dying that was, at least partially, moral driven and embedded in processes of reciprocity and mutual obligation. Yet, while a sense of obligation to at least consider religion or talking to the chaplain did emerge in their stories, it was more complex than a matter of subjugation to normative conceptions of being 'at peace with God'. All interviewees accepted the need for religious supportive care at end of life, just not as a standard aspect of hospice care. For those who did not have religious beliefs or a desire to discuss religion, such pressures may in fact produce existential dilemmas that otherwise would not have emerged. This represents a key example of the hospice as precariously placed between the care of the body and the care of the soul.

## Discussion

Despite the recognition that the institutionalisation of dying is fundamentally changing the experience of dying for many people, virtually no research has hitherto been done to explore dying in hospices from a sociological perspective: how the lived experience of dying is shaped by specialist institutions taking an increasingly dominant role; what options the institution offers those who choose (or otherwise) to die away from the home; and, what forms of constraint, liberation and power emerge from the institutional moralities that have emerged within palliative and hospice care practices?

The participants' accounts shed significant light on some of these issues including their sense of (restricted) autonomy and concerns around the right to choose within the hospice. While there was acknowledgement that the hospice came with baggage (for example, 'you don't get to die your way') and distinct benefits (for example, 'no-one sees you at your worst') there was a sense of impotency once one had submitted to the organisational principles of 'dying well'. While it is not argued here that individual autonomy is denied or non-existent in the hospice, it seems clear that autonomy becomes more relationally negotiated (situated within the values of staff, carers and family) (Broom and Adams 2010) and thus mediated by moral codes of obligation and reciprocity (Kellehear 2008). Euthanasia or assisted dying and desire for death were not viewed by hospice staff as coherent or commensurable with the hospice model of care and remained largely unspoken about. Instead of viewing such 'utterances' (Johansen et al. 2005) from patients as authentic desires to end their life, they were viewed as a 'call for help' from the hospice staff.

Religious support was often viewed as a resource to assist those 'calling for help' through assisting dying requests. Yet, the accounts presented reveal how religious guidance in the hospice produces a range of emotions and interactive processes that are worthy of significant sociological investigation. The chapel, chaplain and religious 'talk' was calming and therapeutic for some while concurrently anxiety provoking or irrelevant for others (see also Edmondson et al. 2008; Exline and Yali 2000). Several of the participants felt that in providing a chapel and chaplain the hospice was breaching the boundaries between individual belief versus formalised care. Ultimately, the religious and political positioning of the hospice was viewed as heavily shaping staff views on euthanasia or assisting dying and 'dying well'.

Sociologically, this positions the hospice as a highly political and morally-laden organisational setting. While all organisational entities are bound by culture, politics and social expectations, unlike most other sites of medical care, the hospice contains, employs and espouses explicit values about the existential. It actively involves, encompasses and often literarily accommodates stakeholders (for example, family members and carers) in very different ways to an in-patient hospital environment. The hospice is thus a highly interactional and negotiated setting where complex combinations of grief, celebration, pain and joy are interactionally enacted and expressed. Such interpersonal dynamics necessarily support and demand the moral practices of gift, obligation and reciprocity (Broom and Cavenagh 2010, 2011).

The moral codes, in the context of the hospice, may be viewed as emerging from cultural constructions around the 'untimely death' (Parry 1982, 1994). The participants' experiences are an illustration of how organisations, such as hospices, can be complicit in the production and governance of such ideas. Their stories reveal a tension between a desire for a swift death vis-à-vis the organisational governance of 'timely deaths' (cf. Payne, Langley-Evans and Hillier 1996). The idea of 'timely' (or untimely) deaths relates to the politics of human dignity in modern nation states – a code of rights that also encompasses ideas about honour, respect and glory. Such moral codes form the bedrock of the constitutional democracies of Western civilisation.

To take a step back for a moment, there are dual processes evident in the accounts presented here. The first is a moral economy of dying (see Booth 1994) that provides a relational framework for 'dying well', through cultural scripts around 'good deaths' and ideas about gift and obligation. Intimately intertwined with quasi or explicitly religious notions of 'closure', 'acceptance' and 'a natural end', this morality of dying produces interpersonal dilemmas, dilemmas about a responsibility to live as long as one can (see also Broom 2009a), responsibility to reconcile existential questions before death, and responsibility to accept one's end. The second concurrent process is the governance of timely deaths (Parry 1982, 1994), human dignity and the universally recognised right to life. In the context of dying in a hospice, such rights are manifest within the organisational governance of the 'unnatural' or 'untimely death', of which euthanasia/assisted dying may be viewed as a part. Such moral codes are anchored in the writings of social contract theorists such as Hobbes and Rousseau (Hobbes 1670; Rousseau 1973), that is, a universally ascribed social contract or promise of life that the modern state is obliged to provide. Social 'contracts' as evident in this setting both allow certain possibilities and limit human agency. The hospice thus represents the bureaucratisation (James and Field 1992) of the 'timely death' buttressed by a religiously framed transitional mode of 'exit' from this world. Religious supportive care – and various religious rationalities around suffering and acceptance – provide one resource for making sense of, and coping with, suffering in the absence of an assisted or self-determined end.

Ultimately, the revealing of the hospice as religiously, culturally and morally bound does not limit its value in contemporary end-of-life care. Rather, my aim here has been to situate the hospice more clearly in cultural, political and social context and examine how it may be shaping contemporary experience of dying. Theoretically, further work is needed around the social and organisational expectations in and around dying in a hospice. In an increasingly globalised and eclectic cultural landscape, end-of-life care providers will need to be responsive to a widening range of cultural, religious and moral codes. Revealing current alignments, politics and normative institutional practices is the first step in supporting such organisational adaptation. I move now to a focus on another key site of moral exchange and relations of obligation, that of kinship and the dynamics of family at the end of life.

# Chapter 5
# Families and Dying

## Introduction

As outlined in Chapters 3 and 4, dying involves a range of important moral performances and relational dynamics which may function to allow and disallow certain things within the process of dying. This is captured in the well-established literature on the social construction of 'the good death' (Hart, Sainsbury and Short 1998) or the more contemporary notion of the 'good enough death' (McNamara 2004). Such discursive practices that codify the 'best way to go' have emerged from a range of cultural dispositions around suitable ways of dying and caring for the dying. These sociocultural scripts are concurrently enabling, as well as being restrictive and normative in their effects (Chattoo and Ahmad 2008; McPherson, Wilson and Murray 2007). My approach in this book is to expose the cultural scripts and social practices surrounding dying as worthy of ongoing consideration in terms of how they create opportunity and constraint in end-of-life care settings – rather than to demonise them. I hope this will facilitate ongoing questioning of how we die, why we die in these particular ways, and what other forms of dying may be possible.

I turn now to focus on *the family* and how dying is *relationally* experienced, achieved and resisted in relation to kinship ties. I explore how recent shifts in family structures and family life may be reflected in, and inflect, the contemporary experience of dying. While I have already touched on the relational and intersubjective character of dying in previous chapters – particularly relations between professionals and patients – there are also important kinship ties and relations of informal care which are crucial to gaining a full understanding of dying as a truly social occasion (Aoun et al. 2005; Christ and Blacker 2005; Clark et al. 2006). The family, in all its forms, is a critical social structure in shaping individual and collective experiences of dying, and with its constantly shifting and diversified forms, offers an evolving relational influence at the end of life (Goldberg 2010; Kellehear 2008). Whether supporting formalised in-patient hospice or specialist palliative care or providing intensive informal end-of-life care in the home, families and informal carers are critical to the social practice of dying, and the perpetuation, rejection and reframing of the moral and political underpinnings of the dying process (Grande, Addington-Hall and Todd 1998; Kellehear

2008). Families themselves are exposed to problematic cultural normativities around *responsibility* for the dying person and gendered expectations around care (Fine 2007). Thus, the family is a vitally important 'unit of analysis' and a critical player in the social production of dying (see also Hudson and Payne 2011; Harding and Higginson 2003; Hudson, Remedios and Thomas 2010; King and Quill 2006; Kramer, Boelk and Auer 2006).

The centrality of the family in achieving successful 'outcomes' within palliative and hospice settings has been well documented within the health and medical literature (King and Quill 2006; Nebel 2011). Recognition the critical role of the family involvement in dying has led many to argue for the family to be the 'unit of care' in palliative care contexts rather than the individual patient (Nebel 2011; see also Aoun 2004; Goldberg 2010; Grande et al. 2009; Harding and Higginson 2003; McMillan et al. 2006; Thomas, Morris and Harman 2002). This has become an idealised model of care for many working in palliative care. While a family-directed model has the potential to subsume the dying individual's needs within the broader family unit, among other shortcomings, 'treating' and 'caring' for an individual who is dying as an isolated entity neither works particularly well, nor reflects the reality of how things are done by clinicians (Stajduhar et al. 2010). The dying process is necessarily relational and involves input from a plethora of stakeholders, desires and influences. Care strategies and trajectories thus require input from a range of formal and informal care providers as well as the individual who is dying (Nebel 2011).

Because of this relationality, dying can produce significant tension around individual desires and family values and needs. The character of end-of-life care is often deeply embedded in family expectations and cultural ideas around duty and mutual responsibility. This has led to end-of-life care providers acknowledging the reality that 'managing families' and interpersonal relations must be a key consideration in the delivery of care (Goldberg 2010, Grande et al. 2009, Hudson and Payne 2011). In many cases entry into an in-patient palliative care or hospice unit may be about the increasingly high demands placed on individual families and their lack of capacity to cope at home (Clark et al. 2006, Harding and Higginson 2003). In such contexts, family dynamics (that is, closeness, discord and all those dynamics in between) can strongly mediate everything from place of death to the point of entry into formal care, and ultimately, the dying process.

While families can be critical to 'successful deaths', they can in turn be influential in 'difficult deaths' (Goldberg 2010; Grande et al. 2009; Nebel 2011). Clearly, categorisations such as these are highly dependent on one's subject position. Perhaps more concerning, the economic capacity of families to provide informal care is increasingly differentiated, creating an environment of significant inequity in capacity to support 'good enough deaths'. Place of death becomes not simply about personal or family preference, or even individual choice, but rather the capacity to care (or be cared for) in informal settings, a situation strongly tied to economic capability and resources.

The issue of equity relates also to how recent changes in family structures and social expectations (Beck and Beck-Gernsheim 1996; Beck and Beck-Gernsheim 2001) have shifted what occurs at the end of life. The more extensive use of public and private specialist in-patient hospice care in Australia and internationally, may be closely connected to the (decreasing) capacity of working families to support the dying process through informal care. Access to formal care provision at the end of life will increasingly be restricted to those with private insurance cover with the privatisation of specialist palliative care.

As suggested in previous chapters, for previous generations, dying and being cared for at home by family was largely taken for granted. This notion of dying as necessarily taking place in the home and supported purely by family continues to change as hospices and specialised in-patient palliative care services shape the range of options for care and the stakeholders involved at the end of life (Broom and Cavenagh 2010). Given changing cultural and economic influences, the responsibilities of the immediate and extended family and those of the state at the end of life may be shifting considerably.

The dying process is thus situated within a dynamic social and cultural environment whereby the very character of family and family life is evolving. Intergenerational relationships have changed over the last few decades with improvements in life expectancy, and increasing fluidity in familial relationships across the life span (Silverstein and Giarrusso 2010) reconfiguring family typologies (Strong, DeVault and Cohen 2010). Just as family life changes and presents challenges in the contexts of social welfare, parenthood and so on, so too do such changes present challenges for the end-of-life experience. We know little about the interplay of the family and experiences of dying. In this chapter I explore experiences of 'the family' in the last few weeks of life, as recounted by hospice in-patients themselves.

## Background

### *Families and Informal Care at the End of Life*

A family member entering palliative and end-of-life care settings significantly impacts on families and informal carers, and for the majority of people, a family member dying is *the* most significant event in their lives. Families and informal carers carry a significant proportion of the burden of dying, but also gain from the experience of caring for the dying (such as, personal growth, reconnection, acts of giving and gift, relief and so forth). For many people dying engenders positive relational experiences, for both 'patient' and 'carer'. However, it is also clear that families and informal carers often struggle through the dying process and have unmet needs (Grande et al. 2009; Goldberg, 2010; Harding and Higginson 2003; McMillan et al. 2006; Thomas, Morris and Harman 2002). This has led to the development of a sociology of informal care, as well as a more health services oriented exploration of the role of informal carers and families in end of life settings (Olson 2012; see also Aoun et al. 2005; Clark et al. 2006; Hudson, Aranda and Kristjanson 2004; Hudson and Payne 2011; Hudson, Remedios and Thomas 2010; Kristjanson and Aoun 2004). This has included work on clinicians' interactions with families and caregivers (Christ and Blacker 2005) and practice-driven strategies to support families more effectively in clinical contexts (King and Quill 2006; Kristjanson and Aoun 2004; Redinbaugh et al. 2003; Walsh et al. 2007). There has also been some research on family decision-making and interpersonal dynamics (for example, Kramer, Boelk and Auer 2006; Winter and Parks 2008) which has illustrated the potential for conflict and emotional difficulties when negotiating end-of-life decisions, including disagreements over discontinuing treatment and deciding the place of death. The data has been largely clinically-driven rather than sociologically driven (Seale 1998a), and has focused on the perspectives from stakeholders other than people who are themselves dying (Nebel 2011). In my hospice fieldwork I was interested in successes and tensions or conflicts within the family from the perspectives of hospice patients themselves. I explore these reflections in the section below.

### *Changing Family Structures, Cultural Shifts and Families at the End of Life*

Family dynamics at the end of life reflect wider cultural practices in and around kinship and collectivist versus individualist culture (Riley 1983; Seale 1998a). Thus, in exploring families in the in-patient hospice setting it is important to consider the cultural production and experiences of families more broadly (Strong, DeVault and Cohen 2010), and how cultural forces are involved in the shaping of dying as a social and relational process (Kellehear 2008; Howarth 2007b; Seale 1998a). In many respects the emergence of the hospice movement and the formalisation of palliative care as a medical speciality (Clark 2007) have taken place concurrently with a significant shift in family values and structures in the mid to late twentieth century. Changes include increasing diversity in the family form and interpersonal ties, increasing precariousness of conjugal relationships, shifts in family divisions of labour and changes in the style and geography of extended kin networks (Beck and Beck-Gernsheim 2001; Giddens 1991; Smart 2007).

These changes have not been explored in detail in relation to experiences of dying and end-of-life care, even though the responsibility of family or community, caring and dying are now considered (at least in part) as situated within the realm of the state and increasingly the private sector (James and Field 1992, see also Fine 2007).

Biomedical orientations toward (individualised) physiological control, at least initially in the development of palliative medicine, resulted in a largely patient-centred model of end-of-life care, rather than a family-centred view. But 'family-centred care' remains an ideal rather than a grassroots reality (Goldberg 2010; Grande et al. 2009; Hudson and Payne 2011). To some extent the in-patient palliative unit or hospice provides a means of placing the dying person 'in care' and although often a clinical necessity rather than an individual or family decision it can potentially reduce the burden on the family (McPherson, Wilson and Murray 2007, Nebel 2011). However, entry into an in-patient palliative care or hospice unit also poses new questions and complexities around family relations and intergenerational care. These include the problematic of the diversities in family dynamics, the potential shift in perception of responsibility for caring, and the capacity of the specialised palliative and hospice units to provide care that is responsive to varying family needs and desires. Therefore I argue for a relationally-located conceptualisation of dying within an in-patient palliative care and hospice environment.

## *Understanding Dying as Relational and Embedded in Family Dynamics*

Dying is a collective rather than individual experience and a space infused with complex agendas, needs, desires and interpersonal dynamics (Kellehear 2008; Howarth 2007b; Seale 1998a; Stajduhar et al. 2010). It is culturally located within a particular level of socio-economic development, cultural expectations and intergenerational relations (Hales, Zimmermann and Rodin 2008; Kellehear 2008; Howarth 2007b; Grande, Addington-Hall and Todd 1998; Seale 1998a). Intergenerational ideas about collective as opposed to individual responsibility (including the state versus the family) *may* be increasingly mediating experiences and family dynamics at the end of life. I draw on Giddens's (1991) concept of ontological security and Beck and Beck-Gernsheim's (2001) notion of individualisation to provide a novel lens for beginning to explore how families shape the end of life in an in-patient hospice. My aim in this chapter is to develop a critical analysis of how family structures and values may shape end-of-life care and the wider social production of dying (Broom and Cavenagh 2010; Chattoo and Ahmad 2008; Kellehear 2008; Sivaramakrishnan 2005).

## Into the Field

### *The Strains on Families*

Once again, I draw on interviews and my ethnographic work with in-patients in the last few weeks of life receiving care in a hospice New South Wales, Australia. Another key theme in the interviews in addition to those explored in the previous chapters, was the impacts on family and/or carers of being in the hospice. While this issue has been explored from various stakeholder perspectives previously (cf. Aoun et al. 2005; Clark et al. 2006; Redinbaugh et al. 2003; Thomas, Morris and Harman 2002; Walsh et al. 2007), rarely has there been an opportunity to explore this issue from the perspectives of hospice in-patients themselves. We know that family pressures, conflicts and interpersonal dynamics can be perceived very differently depending on the particular stakeholder consulted (child, father, brother, carer, clinician) (Aoun et al. 2005; King and Quill 2006), yet few have consulted hospice in-patients themselves as they have been generally considered to be too burdened by the dying process. However, such interpersonal and intergenerational complexities may actually be crucial to understanding and improving quality of life and supportive care needs (Broom and Cavenagh 2010; see also Hudson and Payne 2011). As shown in the following quotes, home versus hospice decisions are often embedded in considerations as to the family coping regardless of patient preference:

> *Participant* (female): I would prefer to be at home. Um, but then again, by the same token, if hubby doesn't think he can cope, which, it may come to that point, where he can't cope, with the whole physical thing, the mental thing of me being at home, then I will willingly come in [again].

Another participant comments:

> *Participant* (male): Of course I would rather be at home but it isn't just about me is it?

Another participant comments:

> *Participant* (male): Yeah, my biggest problem or concern is that when I get home how is [wife] going to handle me, you know?

As shown above, and in many of my other participants' accounts, the admission to the hospice was almost unanimously viewed as a product of families' (and often patients') inability to manage complex symptoms, pain and suffering in the home setting. While feelings about this transition and the move to the hospice were complex and differentiated across the interviewees' accounts, an underlying theme was the guilt of being a burden on the family as a whole *combined with* a sense of uncertainty as to whether moving to the hospice was in fact 'giving up'. A stoicism–burden dynamic was clearly evident in their accounts in that moving to the hospice was presented as concurrently regressive (closer to death and alienating) and relieving (less of a burden on the family). Moreover, once in the hospice itself, there was a trauma of disease progression ('people watching me go downhill') as well as a sense of opportunity ('a chance to make things right'):

> *Participant* (female): Yes, definitely, I do [worry about my family]. Because they're, living alone, they've watched me go downhill.

As mentioned above, while the (often) swift disease progression of the hospice stage was distressing, it was also viewed as a key time to 'making things right' and thus held both positive and negative emotions for the participants and their families:

> *Participant* (female): It's a very hard thing to wait to die, and to see the affect [sic] that it has on your family and those around you. It's good in a way, because you can do things. You can, mend fences, you know … I've helped my kids now [financially] rather than waiting until I'm dead. That's good, you can do all that and feel good that you've done it … But watching them, watch you, decline and die, I can't image what that's like. Because I'm not them, I'm me, I can't imagine how they feel and it's not, it's not pleasant. It really isn't, if there was some other way that you could do it. If you could do both, you know, get all your fences mended and do everything you want to do, and then have a heart attack and go quickly, that would be the ideal thing. But, it will never be. But I don't know, I worry about him [my husband], I worry about them all, but there's nothing that I can do.

Given that the majority of the participants had advanced cancer and thus potentially faced a drawn out death (versus a sudden heart attack or 'a quick death'), the dying process was viewed as concurrently cruel and kind on their families. The hospice stage was talked about as providing opportunities for 'saying goodbye', 'mending fences' and 'tying up loose ends'. Yet, the drawn out death was also viewed as coming at a price for them and their family, and furthermore, as asking too much of some families. Thus, in-patient hospice care was viewed as both difficult but also a solution to the intolerability of suffering in the presence of, or impossible requirements for, families at home:

> *Participant* (male): As I say I can't move from my belly button down. My wife's not a real big person and she's had three hip replacements. I just don't see how she can handle me at home, I really don't, without someone else being there all the time. I'm just too big for her to handle. I'm about six foot one and I weigh, well I did weigh about ninety-five kilos ... And this is my biggest concern, that if I go home and something happens to her, what's going to happen then? It's going to be worse off.

As another participant reflects, much of the sense of potential suffering at home amongst the participants was situated around the dual concerns of maintaining dignity and not frightening the family with 'out of control' symptoms and pain:

> *Participant* (male): It's just, going with a little bit of dignity, not in a mess, not lying in a nappy full of, shit, for want of another word, and not being a frightening sight to those that are sitting there, maybe watching me, you know, sort of thing. They [family] want it to be peaceful for me, but I want it peaceful for them [family] as well, and at least I know, with the Palliative Care Service will try to do as much as they can ...

This excerpt reflected a common narrative within the interviews around caring for the family through not exposing them (or the patient themselves) to the indignities of bodily disintegration and lack of bodily control (see Chapter 9 for discussion on 'The Dying Body'). Moreover, talk within the interviews reflected a sense of relief of their relocation to hospice care for their families and the identity-related issues around not wanting 'people to help':

> *Participant* (female): Well, I couldn't get over it. My family just could see that I certainly needed some help, and that was it. They all just surrounded [me] and they've been doing my gardening and cleaning my house, not that the house is dirty with one person in it, but they've been doing all that, doing the washing, and that type of thing. That I haven't had to even hint at it [their struggle], and that's been very good … [but] you don't want people to [help], I've always been one that's helped other people all my life ...

Several participants described admission to the hospice in terms of relieving family caregivers from stress, and improving their capacity to cope emotionally with their loved one's illness:

> *Participant* (female): He's [husband] always been very quiet and sort of laid back, he doesn't really say a lot, and it does bother me sometimes as to whether he's actually coping or not, and that was the reason I said about that going home, about making him not feeling as though he can't cope. Because that's the last

> thing I want for him. If he feels as though he can't cope, I would rather be in here, if that gives him a chance to come here spend some time, and then go home and get his head together … And I do worry about him, because he's not really the sort of person to go out actively looking for help, he'll try and get through it himself.

All participants expressed considerable concern regarding their family's capacity to cope and the broader impact of their dying process on families and relationships. The hospice was often perceived as a solution (albeit limited) to collective suffering and the family's incapacity to cope. The comment 'I would rather be in here, if that gives him a chance to come here spend some time, and then go home and get his head together' encapsulated the experience of the majority of the participants. The hospice represented a lowering of burden on the family given the extensive suffering they had to endure, and their own desire to have positive family interactions rather than push their families to the limit. There was regular commentary around being able to 'send them [family] home' and 'let them keep living'. Yet, despite recognition of the relief the hospice provided, it was also very clear that it could not adequately substitute for home and family intimacies in a 'natural' context:

> *Participant* (female): There's no place like our own home, and I'd rather be at home. I'm not fretting because I'm in here, but I like my home ...

In several other participants' accounts, the hospice was still experienced in largely institutional terms with 'normal' everyday family life in some respects disrupted by the formalised setting. Staff were held in high regard, but the professional, economic and institutional nature of staff–client dynamics in the hospice presented a clear contrast to interpersonal dynamics at home with family. The hospice was perceived to provide relief to families, but also as somewhat lacking in authenticity and intimacy in day-to-day interactions and encounters typical of a community and home setting.

### *Supportive and Amazing Families*

Many deaths do not imbue a sense of resolution, interpersonal closeness and strong family support (King and Quill 2006, McMillan et al. 2006). There is a broad spectrum of family experiences, and such diversities often lack visibility within the academic literature (Aoun et al. 2005). During the interviews I asked participants to talk about their family's responses, reactions and interpersonal dynamics (see also King and Quill 2006). With the relatively small sample there is a limit to the extent to which I can extrapolate from these participants' accounts; rather, I seek to illustrate potential diversities in family responses within the dying process (Aoun et al. 2005, Hudson and Payne 2011) and to capture discord, conflict and tension as well as support and intimacy. As expected, there was no singular family (end-of-life) dynamic; there were no consistent emotions, interactions or reported dynamics indicative of the in-patient hospice family experience. I begin with accounts of the family as (reportedly) highly supportive while in-hospice:

> *Participant* (male): Oh, amazing. I'm blown away, absolutely blown away [by my family], I can't believe how good they've been. Um, but they've been fabulous, just fabulous.
>
> *Interviewer*: And have they got support?
>
> *Participant*: I think if they need it, I think they can access that so I don't think ... the only person who feels sort of slightly isolated from all of this is my daughter, who lives in [city], and it's just a long way away … It's just the distance … and I know that she would like to see me more often, but how do you talk to her, it's just not practical. So, my son, comes up every weekend with his wife and son who lives with his family, and we just sit around and chat for a while and then he goes home again …

In several interviews, participants talked about the extent and importance of support offered by family members:

> *Participant* (female): Amazingly supportive, I've been very lucky … he [husband] spends his whole time here and is amazingly supportive, they [family] all are …

The above excerpts provide examples of the participants' reflections on their highly supportive and close families. Such accounts provide insight into the positive and empowering potential of family structures in providing support during the dying process. The examples highlight the continued relevance of and investment in close family ties, despite emerging cultural emphases on processes of individualisation (Smart 2007).

### *Family Conflict, Feelings of Loneliness and Abandonment*

The interviews revealed the fact that dynamics between family members and the dying person are not necessarily positive and affirming at the end of life. Though participants often expressed shame in telling such stories, family struggles, lack of family support and even an absence of physical presence in the hospice were common. Three participants in particular revealed important examples of family difficulties within in-patient care and at the end of life more generally. For these participants, in-patient care and end-of-life processes had either enhanced existing family discord, or existing issues had carried through to the hospice setting. The 'drawn out death' interplayed with temporal shifts in the support and presence of family members. It is important to note here that some of the participants had entered the hospice as a result of their families' inability to support or cope with the dying process at home. Economic pressures, value of intergenerational relationships, and long-term conflicts were talked about as shaping problematic dynamics:

> *Participant* (female): Um, my son and [his] wife have benefitted from the help that I've had, because they are too busy to spend a lot of time with me. My two daughters, I hardly ever see them, um, it's very, very rare that I see them, because, it all changed when I developed this disease, because I refused to have um, [biomedical] treatment for it. Their attitude towards me changed. They more or less can't be bothered with me anymore … and they just, my two daughters just stay away [from the hospice].

There were also examples of tension and discord between participants and their family members, particularly in perceptions of the extent of support offered by family members:

> *Participant* (male): Well my home arrangements, no … they're not [good] ... [talks at length about specific issues of ongoing conflicts while receiving palliation at home from daughter and son-in-law] … Well, I still get treated like shit, especially from him [son-in-law].

While the majority of participants represented the end of life as a time for families to 'come together' and 'mend fences', these accounts suggest more varied circumstances. Some participants felt they got little or no support from their families, and some perceived that the support and interaction diminished as the dying process continued. The reasons are complex and differ for each person and for each family. And, while further research is needed exploring dynamics across institutions, communities and individual biographies, the interviewees' accounts did indicate that outside pressures (such as, work, mortgages, geographical distance and so on) limited the capacity of their families to 'be there' during the last few weeks of life. Albeit in a minority of cases, families may have such significant ongoing tensions that interaction and communication breaks down entirely. A fairly common account was that family attention (and capacity to support) waned over time, as distance from the initial admission to the hospice increased. As one participant said, 'their lives go on and ours don't'. I would suggest that such dynamics may resonate with recent cultural and structural shifts towards individualisation, where biographies are increasingly characterised by choice rather than tradition or obligation (Beck and Beck-Gernsheim 2001). Although further research is needed, the circumstances talked about by participants may also reflect aspects of Giddens's notion of ontological security (Giddens 1991): the very existence of the hospice and the approach some families take within the dying process reflects broader cultural questioning of ontological security, and the precariousness of previously set out ways to live, and die, in the life trajectory. Ultimately, the complexity and variability of potential end-of-life experiences reveal circumstances where a sense of ontological security or safety in the predictable or the routine is no longer present.

### *Family versus Individual Preferences and Choice*

Much of the family dynamics discussed within the interviews centred on the relationality of dying preferences and the degree to which dying was situated within a dialectic between individual preference and collective desire. The family wanted the person to 'hang around' and 'make the most of it' whereas some participants desired a quick death. Family tensions were commonly situated within this dynamic:

> *Participant* (male): I know [wife's name] wants me to hang around as long as I can. Um, no, I've got no intentions of giving up, I've got every intention of fighting it for as long as I can. Um, you're fighting a losing battle, but what the hell, you've got to be in it! ... My own preference, as I said, would've been to have a sudden death. But, you don't get your preference, you don't get a choice. You get whatever cards were dealt.

For several of the participants, individual preferences or ideals were situated within a consideration of the desires of their family, particularly in circumstances where family members were often present within the hospice. The maintenance of stoicism and to 'fight' for the benefit of family members was frequently revealed as an important element of preserving relationships at a time of considerable tension and stress. Just as the hospice was considered influential in defining the types of ways one should go (that is, acceptance/resolution), so too were families. Often there was talk of families making statements in clinical consultations such as 'you will fight on won't you' or 'he does want to live, don't you', illustrating the ways in which family needs often become part of the person's performativity of the good death (McNamara 2004).

One exception to the family-versus-individual choice dynamic was evident in the case of a male participant with heart failure. This participant spoke at length of his desire to die, and had previously attempted suicide as a way to escape what he viewed as a drawn out death. For this participant, family, in particular his daughters, were highly supportive in that they strongly espoused his right to die, rather than wanting him to 'hang around':

> *Participant* (male): But it's my decision, and I should have been left alone. I do believe this, and I have lots of friends, who my children said that to, "you should have just left him alone. You'll go, you wanted to go. You've had your life".

The above excerpt illustrates an important point in that family desires were not always about encouraging the 'good fight' nor indeed counter to those of the patient. Indeed, families were often strong advocates of patient choice and I seek not to diminish their crucial role here. However, there were also relational aspects which I argue are important for situating their care decisions and broader experiences at the end of life.

## Discussion

This chapter merely scratches the surface of the issues facing families with members in in-patient hospice or specialist palliative care, let alone issues facing families dying across other sites of care. I have touched on some important family dynamics and indicated the extent to which we may need to rethink how families can shape dying in formalised care settings. The interviewees' accounts certainly resonate with existing empirical work in related contexts (for example, aged care and nursing home institutionalisation) that points to the influence and relevance of family and informal carer dynamics (cf. Fisher and Lieberman 1999; McLennon, Habermann and Davis 2010; Noel-Miller 2010). Such studies emphasise the role of family/caregiver characteristics as *related* to those of the patient in shaping trajectories within aged care and the processes of institutionalisation at the end of life. The interviews also highlighted the importance of the *relational* aspects of family caregiving for health promotion in palliative care settings (Stajduhar et al. 2010).

Most evident in participants' accounts was the idiosyncrasy of families, and that a 'one size fits all' approach has no place within frameworks for managing the end of life (King and Quill 2006). Participants each recounted their family's responses to the dying process and caring practices with the expected spectrum which ranged from close-knit families to those who, for one reason or another, were experiencing ongoing conflict and discord. These family dynamics were talked about as heavily shaping the experience of end-of-life care. Problematic dynamics and interpersonal and intergenerational conflicts continued within the dying process. The hospice concurrently was a space with (family) conflicts and divisions, as well as facilitating intimacies and reconnections. The hospice experience was for some an opportunity to reconnect and repair, but for others it reflected disconnections and the sense of loss and alienation. I heard of benevolent and amazing families, difficult and challenging families, and absent ones, even within this relatively small group of hospice patients. These accounts illustrate a diversity often not acknowledged within the delivery of palliative care.

Few social scientists have attempted to link together research on changes in family life and related forms of identity work with the dying process even though the dying process is acknowledged to be culturally located and specific to our particular level of socio-economic development, cultural orientations and recent cultural turns (Glaser and Strauss 1968; Howarth 2007b; Kellehear 2008; Lawton 2000; Prior 1989). These participants' accounts suggest that the dying process may be shaped – sometimes subtly – by intergenerational shifts (enhanced individualisation and uncertainty), potentially raising important questions surrounding cultural ideas about responsibility (of the state versus the family). Specifically, the notion of ontological security (Giddens 1991) may be further explored as a sensitising concept. A person's sense or confidence in their life trajectory and how being exposed to the realities of caring for a family member who is dying may undermine that security (Giddens 1991), not least because it forces reflection on the value of one's own life trajectory, choice biography (Beck and Beck-Gernsheim 2001) and the circumstances of one's own imagined death. Such an idea around shifting cultural forces provides an important lens for further exploring the dilemmas of families and individuals at the end of life. Comments such as 'they are just paying off their mortgage', 'they have no time now they have kids' and 'coming in here was easier than burdening them' were examples of participants' resistance to burdening their families (McPherson, Wilson and Murray 2007) – an embedding of a *perceived* lack of sense of responsibility within the context of contemporary pressures. The participants often talked with me about changing social and economic conditions, particularly in relation to work and family. Yet, close family ties were still strongly evident and thus I suggest that further research is needed to explore the extent to which 'traditional' social influences continue to provide routine ontological security, and the potential impacts on end-of-life processes.

The interviewees' accounts of family life also resonate with Beck and Beck-Gernsheim's (2001) notion of individualisation, that is, the cultural pressures on individuals to create and maintain their own biography based on personal choices rather than structural forces or traditions. Changing social and cultural forces may thus prompt individuals to question the character and meanings of family, caring and dying. Over time, the rights and responsibilities model of caring and dying may be increasingly disrupted (or perhaps transformed) by an increasingly precarious existence *for some* family members. A number of participants reported extremely dedicated and compassionate families and carers who were uncompromising in their support. This augments existing research on the family that emphasises the *persistence* of investment in close personal relationships (see for example, Smart 2007; Jamieson 1998; Gross 2005). However, I argue that broader social, cultural and economic trends associated with processes of individualisation should be further explored in terms of developing an understanding of how families and relationships might be changing. Within the interviews there was often mention of the contemporary disruption of intergenerational responsibility and the hospice played a role in reinforcing caring as negotiable rather than a family obligation. While further work is needed to tease out trends, it is possible that 'traditional' rituals of family caregiving may be undermined by individualised living contexts as well as emotionally reflexive practices (Beck and Beck-Gernsheim 1996). This was evident in the interviews when family members were talked about as unable to adequately perform caring duties and often were constrained by work or immediate family commitments.

I should emphasise that I do not argue that intergenerational change is a priori problematic, nor do I idealise particular forms of family relations. Rather, here I have outlined some potentially emerging patterns in the perceived relations of care. I have also emphasised that the hospice presents a vital mechanism by which carers and family members can be supported in the context of uncontrollable symptoms and other difficulties. It is worth considering the degree to which some 'individualised' families are able to absorb the responsibilities of care, whether neoliberal influences are subtly shifting the politics of care (Fine 2007), and the extent to which the expectation to care for oneself is a self-fulfilling philosophy. By being increasingly responsible for our own care, welfare, and related decisions – our 'do-it yourself' life projects (Beck and Beck-Gernsheim 1996) – it becomes more difficult to provide care to one's immediate and extended family. As work in other areas has shown, the neoliberal nation-state devolves responsibility for 'healthy' citizen's trajectories, but in doing so limits their capacity to care for the older, sicker generations (Fine 2007). Such conclusions are tentative and I emphasise that further research is needed with a range of stakeholders (including family, primary carers and clinicians) and in home and community contexts to provide suitably nuanced and multifaceted understanding of the intersections of family life and the dying process. That said, this research and that of others suggests that the quest for individual autonomy in late modernity (Beck and Beck-Gernsheim 2001) shifts forms of social inter-connectedness, and may impact on geographical mobility, enhancing individual commitments, for example to paid work, as opposed to social responsibilities, namely the caring role. In a western context dying is already considerably marginalised, compared with many cultures where dying is viewed as part of the life cycle and more ritualised or embraced. Such shifts may also further sequester the dying person/body from families.

Further research is now needed to explore the accounts of families and informal carers themselves, and this has been ongoing at the time of writing this book. Given that this chapter focuses on informal care and the family, it is pertinent to move on to a focus on nursing at the end of life. Nurses provide important links between formal and informal care and provide a complex mix of formal and informal forms of care themselves.

# Chapter 6
# Nursing the Dying

While a wide range of health professionals play a role in the transition to palliative and end-of-life care, and in the dying process, a large proportion of care is delivered by nurses. They are often present for critical discussions about futility (Broom et al. 2014a; Kirby, 2014b) and at the bedside during the dying process (Costello 2006). They are central actors, albeit often acting 'behind the scenes', in the different spheres of the end of life (Broom et al. 2014a). Nurses influence everything from acceptance of dying, to people's experiences of the last few hours of their lives. While doctors are often involved at particular times (e.g. establishing medical futility, withdrawing life-prolonging treatment, prescribing pain relief, confirming time of death), nurses spend large periods of time with patients and their family members, often over months or even years, managing transitions from palliation to end of life and then death (Broom et al. 2014a; Kirby 2014b). They attend to physical suffering but also engage in a wide range of emotional, social and spiritual issues, acting as complex jugglers of various forms of sentimental work (Bolton 2001). In this chapter I focus on the peculiarities of the nursing role at the point of futility and the transition to the end of life, with an emphasis on the importance *and* problems associated with this area of nursing work.

The roles that nurses play in dying are multiple and inter-professionally complex (Costello 2006), for example prompting 'medical referrals' to palliative and/or end-of-life care, picking up the pieces of messy transitions to the end of life, and accompanying people by the bedside as they die (Mok and Chiu 2004). These are highly charged and challenging moments in care, requiring high-level interpersonal skills (Sandgren et al. 2006). Yet, research in this area of the nursing role and care for the dying has been limited (Gaydos 2004), meaning that we know very little about how nurses feel and what they experience when they help negotiate futility and thus accompany their patients toward the end of life (Fillion et al. 2007). Given the changes in nursing as a profession, its complex power relations with medicine (Hibbert et al. 2003; Salhani and Coulter 2009), and the considerable investment of nursing in supporting the dying (Kristjanson 2005; Mok and Chiu 2004), it was surprising to me that there had been relatively little critical sociological investigation of nursing in the context of futility and care for the dying. Thus, I was keen to explore how nurses balance their formal and informal roles within hospitals and hospices, and how (and whether) they act as mediators between doctors, patients and families (McSteen and Peden-McAlpine 2006).

One of the key reasons understanding nursing is critical to understanding dying is because the histories of palliative and end-of-life care are intimately enmeshed with the history and evolution of significant nursing figures and the nursing profession (Clark 2007; Du Boulay and Rankin 1984). In the twentieth century, key figures (including Cicely Saunders) in tandem with religious, community and non-profit organisations were critical in championing better care for the dying (Clark 2007). When partnered with the eventual development of palliative care as a medical specialty in its own right, this resulted in better palliative and end-of-life care and the amelioration of suffering for many people. Yet, with the medical profession more broadly still largely focused on disease control and symptomatology, it has often been nursing that has engaged in the dynamics of futility and ameliorating suffering, and has invested significant energy in developing strategies for better care at the end of life. While much has changed with the development and expansion of palliative and hospice medicine (Clark 2007), these historical precedents still stand. Caring for the dying resonates with traditional nursing values of providing comfort, care and ameliorating suffering, more so that with the disease orientation of much medical care (Du Boulay and Rankin 1984; Saunders 2000; Miracle 2008). Given this, the search for the 'good death' is deeply enmeshed in the practice of 'good nursing' (Costello 2006).

Nursing work has undergone significant transformation over the twentieth and now twenty-first centuries. While the traditional ideals of nursing still heavily inflect nursing practice (Hibbert et al. 2003), processes of professionalisation of the role and systematisation of care have significantly changed the character of nursing labour. As the profession evolves, so too does the character of care for the dying and in this chapter I argue that it is important to consider that nursing work does not operate within a vacuum; rather, it is heavily shaped by important historical as well as contemporary social, inter-professional and political forces (Gray 2010; Hibbert et al. 2003; Salhani and Coulter 2009). These forces include contemporary pressure toward task-orientated nursing and the persistent gendered division of labour in healthcare delivery. While the 'traditional values' of nursing may align quite well with caring for the dying, contemporary shifts in the profession may be challenging the very nature of the nursing role in this context (see also Fillion et al. 2007). In this chapter I begin to interrogate these issues. I focus on mapping the nursing role in managing futility and dying, on experiences of inter-professional dynamics, and on the significance and impact of *emotional work* in everyday nursing practice.

## Background

### *Inter-professional Care and Professional Dynamics*

The role of nurses in managing medical futility and caring for the dying is inter-professional in character (Back et al. 2009). Nurses work closely with doctors, allied health professionals and other nursing teams (such as supportive and palliative care nurses). This places them within (and around) a range of approaches to care (Miller et al. 2008; Powell and Davies 2012). Nursing is strongly influenced by inter-professional dynamics and hierarchical structures (Powell and Davies 2012). These boundaries include the articulations of the 'nursing role' vis-à-vis the 'medical role' and what these conceptual *and* enacted distinctions mean for negotiations around treatment and care. Although nursing care tends to orientate toward providing patients and families comfort and support, nurses also act as mediators between medical staff and patients and families during moments of significant anxiety or distress (McSteen and Peden-McAlpine 2006). Time spent with patients often allows nurses to act in a crucial feedback loop between doctor and patient, exposing the potential for disagreement and inter-professional conflict (Swetenham et al. 2011).

Nurses mediate patient views of futility, or their desire to stop life-prolonging treatment, to medical staff, but within this process they also articulate and perform nursing values. This mediation role and enactment of nursing expertise is in turn situated within a dynamic of medical dominance; a process enmeshed in nurses' core involvement in sentimental work (see Strauss et al. 1982).

### *Nurses' Intimate Access and Emotions at Work*

The broader context of intimacy, sentimentality and emotion in nursing work is crucial to understanding the complex roles of nurses in contexts of futility, the transition to palliative care and in the dying process. There is a rich body of work within the social sciences in this area (e.g. Bolton 2001; Henderson 2001; Phillips 1996; Theodosius 2006; see also Hochschild 1979) yet little work to date has focused specifically on emotion and sentimental work related to the dilemmas around treatment futility and the transition to palliative care (Bailey, Murphy and Porock 2011). The nurse–patient relationship commonly involves significant intimacy, touch and emotional engagement, with nurses often accessing suffering, grief and trauma more acutely than medical staff (e.g. Ablett and Jones 2007; Fillion et al. 2007; Sandgren et al. 2006). Being present at the bedside, so to speak, places nurses where the hour-by-hour, day-by-day undulations of disease progression and human suffering are dominant (Morita et al. 2004; Skilbeck and Payne 2003). Within the context of an (often) extended care relationship and the potential transition to palliative care, the nurse–patient relationship holds significant potential for interpersonal and emotional complexities.

Managing and displaying appropriate levels of emotion are core features of the nurse–patient dynamic (Bailey, Murphy and Porock 2011) reflecting a broader recognition of the performance of emotions as a key tool in nursing. Disassociation or lack of emotion can be perceived as lacking professional competence, as does over-identifying with patients and their families. During the transition to palliative and end-of-life care, this balance of emotion (that is, *just enough* but *not too much*) is played out within the production of competent nursing, with nurses grappling with the management of emotions as a nursing skill (Bolton 2001; Froggatt 1998; Sandgren et al. 2006). Nurses thus embark on forms of emotion management (Bolton 2001; Froggatt 1998; McQueen 2004; see also Fillion et al. 2007) and the careful and often precarious balancing of intimacy and nursing professionalism (Phillips 1996).

## *Negotiated and Sentimental Order*

In thinking about the transition to palliative care and nursing care of the dying, it is useful to consider professional roles and identities, and the forms of division and day-to-day enactment of power within the hospital. That is, to capture the role differentiation and important skills of the actors, but also how hospital work is ordered in particular ways to suit the particular actors. Several existing concepts within sociology are useful. These include the notions of *emotional labour* (Bolton 2001; Gray 2010; Henderson 2001; McQueen 2004; Miller et al. 2008; Theodosius 2006; Hochschild 1983), *sentimental work* (Strauss et al. 1982), nursing–medicine relations as a *negotiated order* (see for example, Allen 2001; Svensson 1996), (Strauss et al. 1982) and *medical dominance* (see for example, Salhani and Coulter 2009; Powell and Davies 2012; Sanders and Harrison 2008).

Conceptualising nursing–medicine as a negotiated order (Svensson 1996; Strauss 1978) superseded the concept of the nursing–medicine relationship as one based largely on power imbalance and hierarchy (Friedson 1970) and which posited a 'doctor–nurse game' that enabled the nurse to inform and advise the doctor without challenging his/her position (see Stein 1967). The idea of 'the negotiation' in terms of how things are accomplished in organisations allowed for individual agency *and* structural constraint to interplay in the shaping of inter-professional and organisational dynamics (Strauss et al. 1982). Individual action and organisational constraint operate concurrently within negotiations, and in turn reflect forms of agency, power and resistance. Transitions to palliative care, including professional roles, the healthcare division of labour and even a patient's palliative 'status', can be viewed in this way as the product of complex negotiations, inflected by personalities, subjectivities and interpersonal processes.

It is important to note, as Strauss (1978) argued, that not all aspects of an organisation are continually subject to negotiation. However, negotiations do become prominent where lines of action or roles are uncertain. This dynamic of uncertainty and judgment is clearly manifest in the context of treatment futility and the impending shift to palliative care. Negotiations tend to situate around who will do what, when and how much of particular types of work (that is, manage emotions within the ward). The centrality of the negotiation also means that formal guidelines or organisationally prescribed duties may not actually reflect what is done in nursing and medical work on a day-to-day basis (Svensson 1996). As I argue below, despite primarily being a medical decision to refer a patient to palliative care, doctors and nurses actively and informally negotiate around a patient's medical status. The nurse's role in this negotiation centres on their privileged access to patient experience, emotional engagement and their capacity to accurately gauge the limits (and presence) of suffering.

## Into the Field

### *The Purpose of Nursing in the Transition to Palliative Care*

The data I report on below is drawn from interviews with Brisbane-based Australian nurses in 2013, all of whom worked directly with patients who were reaching the point of futility and were involved in the negotiation of transitions to palliative and end-of-life care. The interviews focused on the nurses' experiences of managing patient transitions from potentially life-prolonging to palliative or end-of-life care. Questions were focused on how nurses approach these complex transitional periods in terms of their interactions with doctors, patients and families and, furthermore, how they experience the shift in philosophy of care. Dialogue tended to orientate toward the dilemmas of managing impending futility, maximising comfort and minimising emotional and physical suffering. I began the interviews with a broad question around what it is like – and what it means – to nurse in the transition to palliative care. The nurses' responses focused on their views on the core values of nursing (such as, alleviating suffering, maintaining dignity and comfort):

> *Participant*: We're trying to relieve their symptoms because we don't want to see them suffering. And you know for most nurses their primary aim is in not seeing a patient suffer if they're dying. It's hard enough that a patient is dying. The best scenario for the nurses is that they die with dignity, and they die peacefully, and they die with family around them if they can. And if there's no family the nurses

> become that family for them…if [death is] inevitable we just got to make it the best death we can for a patient … when we do manage to do that there's a bit of pride in that, that we just made it the best we could. [General Medical Ward]

Another respondent comments:

> *Participant*: Personally, I see we get given a unique opportunity to be involved in somebody's end of life. That's a unique thing because if you tell people that you're a cancer nurse invariably they say, "How do you cope? It must be very sad". I'm sure all oncology nurses have been asked that. My answer to them is, "Yes, it can be sad at times, but we get an opportunity for people to have a good death, and if people have a good death then that's much easier to process than if somebody's had a bad death." [Oncology and Haematology]

Another respondent comments:

> *Interviewer*: What is the nursing role in that [transition to palliative care] context?
>
> *Participant*: Just to support and listen, and a lot of family support. We give a lot of support to partners and kids … It's just the simplest little question, "How's it going? And they always say, "Oh thank god someone's asked me how I'm going!" … And lots of hugs, we give a lot of hugs here. We do! But lots of listening, I think just listening, active listening … and it's just the reassurance. I think when you sit down quietly and just explain it to them, they do get reassurance that they're not going to have a terrible death, someone's going to look after them. [Oncology]

As opposed to a medicalised contrast between pre-palliative and palliative care, the nurses viewed similar principles as applying across both these care contexts; the nursing role was not adapted when a patient was deemed to be no longer suitable for life-prolonging intervention. The nursing philosophy was viewed as consistent across these stages with the shifts being centred on the types of conversations between the nurse and patient and the heightened intensity and importance of spending time to access 'what is really going on', as well as ensuring that fears and anxieties about the future were alleviated. In some respects, the nurses framed caring for the dying as an opportunity to 'be involved in a good death', as one participant articulated it. Nursing skills were viewed as particularly crucial in ensuring this and, perhaps, even more important than in life prolonging contexts. Their accounts held that nursing and suffering were inextricably linked. Rather than reflecting a failing in life-prolonging care, the transition reflected a move towards the core business of nursing work. This transitional period required careful strategies for talking to patients.

## *Talking to Patients about Palliative Care and Dying*

Although formal conversations about the need for palliative care were often initiated and conducted by medical staff, the nurses talked about taking on much of the responsibility of conversing with patients about dying, mortality, questions of hope and the fear of suffering within the dying process. The nurses held that it was *their* skill and responsibility to access what was 'really going on' with patients (that is, the backstage), working through what interviewees talked about as 'denial', 'pretend positivity', 'acting strong for the doctor', family resistance and misunderstandings about the meanings of palliative care. Reframing palliative care as something not to be feared was viewed as a key role of the nurses and involved careful consideration and reassuring language:

> *Participant*: … it's a difficult topic. They [nurses] might get asked difficult questions … because it's a big, we sort of underestimate the impact of it on a patient because we've not been in that position. [General Medical Ward]

Another respondent comments:

> *Participant*: And sometimes resistance from the patients too, because they hear the p-word [palliative] and think it's the end. They see it as a, some patients see it as, "Is there nothing more that can be done for me?" And you see it in their faces, when it's mentioned … devastation. [Oncology and Haematology]

Another respondent comments:

> *Participant*: I do know when people mention palliative care they [patients] get a bit panicky that it's the end stage and they're dying or whatnot. So I think it's in the marketing of, why do we utilise the palliative care? [Radiation Oncology]

Another respondent comments:

> *Participant*: I say, "No, no, no it's not the end of life…" and they say, "But are you telling me I'm dying?" … I say, "It's not the end of the world, you can go into pall care, it's just like a side road sometimes" … You've got to get over that part where they think they're going to die [immediately]. And I mean they are dying, but you know … [Medical Oncology]

The nurses talked about 'putting in the time' to have hard conversations reframing palliative care, and gauging how their patients were coping with their technically life-prolonging treatments. These interactions were often contrasted in the nurses' accounts of doctor–patient interactions, that is, that nurses were more able to delve into the highly emotive issue of futility and the individual (highly personal) capacity to 'keep going'. The nurses consistently talked about patients keeping a 'brave face' when doctors were present, and then later having to pass on accurate information about patients to the doctors through informal conversations:

> *Participant*: … the nurses are there and spend much more time with the patient. The [specialist], if you put the stopwatch on when they come into the room for the length of their consult, it's probably at most on a good day they get five minutes with the patient. And often they control the conversation right from the very beginning … So the opportunity for the patient to discuss it is short. The patient thinks that the [specialist] is busy and they don't want to take up their time, and so they'll have a conversation with the nurse because the nurse is there giving a wash, doing their sponge, giving out tablets, doing the obs … I think nurses just, from a compassion point of view, it's just an easier conversation for them. [Oncology and Haematology]

Another respondent comments:

> *Participant*: I think sometimes the doctor can obviously be rushed and will nip straight in and straight out and the patient will say, "Oh, I forgot to talk to them about stopping treatment … " Like if a patient says, "I'm not really, like, I don't want to tell him that I've had enough, *you* tell him". … When we have the time we'll always go and sit and talk to them. So I think they feel more comfortable with the nurses than they do the doctors because they see us a lot more often, and in a way we're a lot chattier than a doctor. [General Medical Ward]

One of the key dynamics that the nurses observed was the tendency of patients to withhold their feelings and preferences within medical consultations and express these in informal moments with the nurses. The nurses were thereby transformed into doctor–patient mediators, introducing, as I explore below, a series of complex inter-professional dynamics, expressing workplace hierarchies and even resulting in disagreements regarding the course of care. The 'bedside chat' was viewed as a crucial means for accessing patients' perspectives and a considered insight that doctors were unlikely to get. The nurses perceived themselves as having a much better understanding of the patient's true situation and experience, emphasising in turn the strength of the ideology of nurses as patient advocates above all else. Families were an additional key actor within the course toward palliative care and, from a nursing perspective, presented significant challenges and opportunities.

### *Families, Palliative Care and Nursing Work*

Even though the nurses talked extensively about their experiences of interaction with patients (potentially) transitioning to palliative care, each of them emphasised that families were usually the most time-intensive and challenging aspect of nursing during the transition. The nurses viewed themselves as responsible for dealing with family members' emotions on the ward, and accepted the challenge of helping families face the inevitability of medical futility and the need for palliative care:

> *Participant*: I think that's why it's so hard to nurse sometimes because even in the same family you can have someone who's saying, "Give them pain relief," and someone else saying, "Why aren't you giving antibiotics" or "Why aren't you doing this and this and this?" with the active treatment side. So it is, I think it's really tough … You're not just dealing with that patient and their diagnosis. [General Medical Ward]

Another respondent comments:

> *Participant*: I think if you mention the word palliative care to a patient or to a family they assume that they have a week left, two weeks left, and that's the care before they die. I don't think they have an enormous amount of understanding that it can be for their benefit in the way of comfort and pain relief and you know, perhaps not a hospital setting. [General Medical Ward]

Another respondent comments:

> *Participant*: Probably I think the biggest thing is the family. That conversation, you know those conversations and level of understanding between, with the families generally with what's happening … I think that, particularly when it becomes futile, the relationship between the nurse and the patient often becomes a relationship with the nurse, the patient and the family … And it's quite hard, we make sure we round [up] all the families and make sure that they're okay and if there's anything they need … sometimes you let them know that it's okay to say goodbye … we have relatives saying, "How long is it going to be? She's been struggling on" and then you'd ask the question, like, "Have you told her it's okay to let go?" [General Medical Ward]

As shown in these excerpts, and in the other interviews, family interactions and dynamics heavily influenced the experience of nursing at the point of futility and transition to palliative care. Albeit through an informal system of maintaining sentimental order within the ward (Svensson 1996; Strauss 1978), the nurses were given the job of 'managing' families, including resolving differences in opinion between family members and the 'overflow of emotions', as one participant stated, around referral to palliative care and dying. Although the medical staff were talked of as interacting with families formally, it was informal nursing where the majority of the work was perceived to be done: the everyday, personal interactions that involved clarification of medical status, grief counselling, dispute resolution and other core emotional skills. These duties and skills were viewed as being part of the nursing role – managing the sentimental order within the ward – yet they were also core to the broader emotional toll of nursing at this point of futility and the transition to palliative care.

### The Emotional Toll of Nursing

The performance of emotions of nursing has been well documented (Bailey, Murphy and Porock 2011; Fillion et al. 2007; Miller et al. 2008; McQueen 2004; Morita et al. 2004; Theodosius 2006) and so too have the emotional impacts of nursing work in palliative and end-of-life care (Ablett and Jones 2007; Fillion et al. 2007; Sandgren et al. 2006; Skilbeck and Payne 2003). It remains a complex issue given the dual issues of doing emotional work and coping with emotions-at-work (Theodosius 2006). What is clear within the existing social science literature is that nurses are heavily involved in working with emotions, and that emotional intelligence is an important nursing skill (McQueen 2004; see also Henderson 2001). Emotions, as they emerged in discussion within the interviews, are concurrently viewed as a resource, a skill and an impediment within nursing. The nurses talked consistently about the impact of the decision to introduce palliative care:

> *Participant*: ... there is an emotional impact of looking after palliative patients or transitioning patients, you know it's a disappointing situation for everyone, particularly the families. You've got all those stages of grief that you have to deal with. Whereas … the doctors come in and they may spend … five minutes or ten minutes or however long, the nurses are there 24/7 and so they're right in the face of everything the patient's going through and their families. And it's often very, very hard on the nurses ... [General Medical Ward]

Another respondent comments:

> *Participant*: Nurses are expected to suck it up, and "it's part of your professionalism and just get on with it". There's no debriefing, there's no access to formal support in that regard … We don't have any bereavement counselling … it's just

> not seeing that as a priority and yet we burn our nurses out … you can just walk out of a place where somebody has just died and then have to go to the beep beep machine and stick up another bag of chemotherapy without having time to even give yourself five minutes to absorb what you've just been part of? … That's the reality on the ward every day… [Supportive/Palliative Care]

Another respondent comments:

> *Participant*: ... I think [you have to be] someone who has a good understanding, who is sympathetic but not overly passionate about what they do. Because I think if they become overly passionate you lose focus and then everything becomes a tragedy and you take on board too much. I think you've got to be able to separate yourself from the patients and their pain, but still provide them with the comfort to actually get them through. You start taking on board their stuff you burn out very quickly… And we've all tipped over the edge. We've all gone too far and taken that one patient in or whatever that is you know, you let your guard down and there's that one patient that's jumped the barrier so to speak, you know? … [Medical Oncology]

The nurses were clear on the challenge of managing their emotional composure despite significant variation between nurses in terms of how they responded emotionally to patient transitions (more on this below). The nurses perceived themselves as asked to do an unrealistic amount of emotional work despite having little if any emotional support themselves. The precariousness was emphasised, with the majority talking about the importance of strict rules around interpersonal connections and effective boundaries, yet also having these 'broken down' in the context of particularly close relationships. Others, although a minority, talked about managing emotions easily and 'not getting involved':

> *Participant*: I don't get too close to my patients … I've always had the view of, you know, everyone says it's amazing to be in the presence of someone when they start their life. And I think it's the same with someone who passes away. That if you were in that situation then you would want the best care you could have … So I'll always keep the conversation professional if I'm in there and talk to them, whether they can hear me or not, let them know what I'm doing, just be very respectful. And I will do the same after they've passed away, I'll still talk to them you know, when I'm cleaning them and taking them downstairs … it doesn't impact me too much to be honest … I'm not sad by it, not affected, I just leave it here at work. [General Medical Ward]

Another respondent comments:

*Participant*: … You've got to be able to distinguish between [your family] that [the patient], it's quite difficult sometimes to pull yourself back, and this is why it's important to have regular days off, to have outside interests, but to not have outside interests that involve patients … They're not your friend so to speak. [Medical Oncology]

It was clear from the interviews that the emotional toll of nursing during the transition was bound by both 'the nursing role' but also individual personalities, idiosyncrasies and professional survival strategies:

*Participant*: Always making sure that there's just that little bit of space between [you and them]. But it's hard not to sometimes … And there's been so many that have meant so much to you. And there'll always be some that break that barrier. You can't pretend that there's not … I've learned it along the line, that there is… just that little something that you just can't give of yourself. That just makes it just that little bit professional. Because there will be someone else tomorrow. [Supportive Care]

Another respondent comments:

*Participant*: The caring's the easy part. I think what's really hard is after you've done that, and you go rushing to a finance meeting and you think, "I haven't got that [report] ready." And I think, "Oh bugger. I'm not on top of that." And that's the risk of [not] getting that balance right … [Neuro-Oncology]

The emotional impacts on nursing and nurses were also viewed as shaped by a perceived lack of preparedness for palliative and end-of-life issues in nursing training:

*Participant*: I hadn't had any palliative care experience. I never did a palliative care prac, so I found it a bit overwhelming at first … I remember in uni we did a little bit on death and dying and how we would feel about it, but I think the theory's a lot different to actual practice.

*Interviewer*: Tell me how?

*Participant*: I think just even being there when someone dies it's so, it's such a different experience than to read about it in a textbook of how you would deal with it and so forth. I think to actually be there and to be around the family and friends and whoever's there at the time, I think to watch their response is definitely a bit more overwhelming. [General Medical Ward]

The emotional toll along with the emphasis on the nurse's role as entailing significant emotional work was talked about by each of the participants as particularly difficult when managing patients and their families through transitions to palliative care. However, despite the complexities, nurses ultimately situated themselves as central to such forms of care and treatment within the hospital. Although incredibly difficult, maintaining sentimental order and the management of emotions (their own as well as their patient's and their families') remained a key responsibility of the nurse within the negotiated order of the hospital.

### *Doctor–Patient Communication, Inter-professional Dynamics and Nursing*

In managing the transition to palliative care, patient care is largely team-based, meaning that interactions between patients and different team members become crucial for each person's role and patient interactions. The nurses talked consistently about the crucial influence of the way medical specialists talked to patients about palliative care and the dying process. These moments were viewed as fundamental in the patient–nurse relationship and patients' experiences of the transition:

> *Participant*: … it all swings on the physician conversations. And how the physicians have communicated with the patients … it can be a whole lot better if the physician is just really honest and upfront with the patient. You know, some of them do it beautifully, but some of them don't do it at all because it's a hard conversation to have, and that makes it really hard for the nurses. You know, sometimes we've got patients who you know have metastatic disease, absolutely zero chance of survival, and yet we are still doing active treatments. And that just sends a very conflicted message to the patient. [General Medical Ward]

Another respondent comments:

> *Participant*: … they [the patient] would have the conversation with the doctor and then they [the patient] would probably stay longer with the nurse and the nurse would go back … and just say, "Well how do you feel about that? How did that go? Did you really understand what the doctor was saying … so if there were issues or they were unsure about it the nurses would just sit with them and guide them around that and pull the doctor back in and say, "Look, I don't really think the message got across." [Radiation Oncology]

Another respondent comments:

*Participant*: So the way it tends to happen around here is the oncologist or the haematologist comes in with very little tact often, delivers bad news, paints a very grim picture of things and then says palliative care will come and see you. So, often the first consultation you have with the patient they're like a deer in the headlights, "Oh my god, palliative care are here, I've been told it's all bad news you know, what's the next step?" And you're sort of backpedalling…it's presented [by the doctor] as a choice to the patient, as if "you've failed" you know? [Palliative Care]

Another respondent comments:

*Participant*: I think partly because some [specialists] don't like talking about death, like it's not part of a conversation that they probably have the comfort to have or the skills to have…That's a much easier conversation. I think sometimes it just comes down to the [specialists] just doesn't know how to do it. [Oncology and Haematology]

Although these nurses' accounts of doctors' approaches to communication about palliative care were quite varied, there was a consistent view regarding the difficulties faced due to the regular occurrence of poor communication in clinical settings. Nurses, as they recounted, are expected to 'mop things up' following short and sometimes abrupt interactions between specialists and their patients:

*Participant*: I walk a bit of a fine line, because while I fully support pall care, and believe in it, [my specialist] does but to a point, [but] he's not ready to get pall care involved as early as I am … I guess we see things differently, he and I. Because I know the families and know the relatives and know what's going on probably in a lot more detail than he does. I think I probably recognise the need earlier. And also I think some doctors take it as a bit of an insult that they have to get palliative care involved, like they've not been successful and they haven't done their job well enough. Part of it is probably ego as well. They're the best person for the job and they know the patient … but they don't know every aspect as well as [nurses]. So yeah, I certainly push for them [palliative care] to be involved, but I can only push so much. [General Medical Ward]

Another respondent comments:

*Participant*: … nurses will harass the doctors basically … I think the goal for the nurses when we palliate is to make it a good death if we can … All nurses should be able to say it [that they need palliation], but not all nurses are confident

> enough to say it. So we escalate … [up the nursing hierarchy]. Nobody, no nurse wants to see a patient distressed. [General Medical Ward]

Another respondent comments:

> *Participant*: I think it's easy if the doctor's kind of agreeing with you and is on your side. It's the moment when they're like, "No, no, no, I'll just manage this. I'll do this, this and this" and, "No we don't need palliative care! Why do we need palliative care?" And you're kind of like, "Actually, this is why. You've done a great job here, and I'm thinking potentially we could move on, the patient's really needing this." [Neuro-Oncology]

A key distinction of the nursing role from the participants' perspectives was an ability to acknowledge futility, and notice (and act upon) patient distress. In this way, the nurses viewed themselves as ideally placed to advocate on behalf of the patient to the specialist who was perceived as being much more focused on the clinical aspects of life-prolonging care as opposed to psycho-social and supportive care. The nurses talked frequently about the inter-professional tensions manifest in the referral to palliative care, both in terms of timing of referral and communication with patients and their families. Professional status was a factor in nurse–doctor communication, with all of the nurses positioning themselves as holding some degree of concern as to how doctors might react to patient advocacy and/or aggressive or explicit prompting of palliative care referrals. What was clear, however, was the centrality of the nurse as patient advocate above all else and the interprofessional cost that this can incur in everyday nursing work.

## Discussion

Within sociology we have seen several key analyses of the transformation of nursing as a profession, and the politics and practices of distinction within the context of nursing compared with medical work and the medical role (Allen 2001; Bolton 2001; Henderson 2001; Strauss et al. 1963; Strauss et al. 1982; Svensson 1996). Here I have expanded on this literature through exploration of nursing accounts of their practice within the negotiation of futility, transition to palliative care and in their care for the dying. I aimed to develop a better understanding of negotiations around palliative and end-of-life care and the extent to which these are situated within particular interpersonal and inter-professional dynamics, and to better understand the interplay of nursing practice and social relations of hope, resistance and futility, unpacking how nurses negotiate their work, roles and the interpersonal complexities.

Following Strauss (1978), key questions for me were what types of work are being done at the point of futility and transition to the end of life and what are the implications for various actors? What emerged was nursing expertise as centred on accessing the backstage of patient experience (that is, 'What is really going on?' and 'How they are really coping?') to assess whether palliative or end-of-life care may or may not be required or topicalised on the ward. Nurses, as revealed in the interviews, are expected to draw on nurse–patient intimacy to facilitate clinical pathways, including establishing whether palliative care is required and informally explaining what palliative care is. The real challenge of this dynamic lay in the complexities of achieving the necessary interpersonal intimacy whilst doing 'technical nursing' and maintaining professional distance. Somewhat paradoxically, interpersonal connectivity was seen as *a resource* and emotional distance as a *professional skill.* In this way the special nursing–patient relationship and privileged access to patient experience concurrently represented organisational and professional *capital* and *difficulty*.

From the participants' perspectives, the nursing role rested firmly on patient and family advocacy and delivering supportive care early and effectively. This also involved ensuring a sentimental order within the ward whereby emotions were kept at manageable levels for various stakeholders including doctors, patients and families. In taking up the role of *intimate* mediators, the nurses were often presented with significant conflicts in philosophy and perspective, particularly in relation to the need for palliative care vis-à-vis the pursuit of decreasingly efficacious life-prolonging options. This negotiated order (cf. Svensson 1996) on one level worked. The nurses recounted intimate connections and of reinserting the importance of patient perspectives and desires into clinical pathways. However, at times they also considered themselves entrapped within a medical–nursing hierarchy whereby they had clear awareness of the need for palliative care, yet palliative status was not forthcoming from a medical perspective. Thus, although the nurses talked about privileged access to patient need and suffering – and prompting early palliative care referrals – they also recounted the persistence of medical dominance within their clinical work and the organisational limits of nursing knowledge in shifting a patient's 'medical status' (cf. Svensson 1996; Strauss 1978).

It is worth considering the implications of nurses orchestrating sentimental order within the ward, that is, the implications of their particular position within negotiations around potential futility and the need for palliative care. As outlined above, they were active in reframing palliative care or 'undoing' what they described as the sometimes abrupt or insensitive communication of some doctors (what Strauss et al. (1982) called *rectification work).* They talked about supporting vulnerable patients experiencing emotional breakdown (what Strauss et al. (1982) called *composure work).* Such examples reflect the role of nurses maintaining the sentimental order of the hospital and at the point of transition. But this role comes with implications and was experienced in conflicted terms by the nurses interviewed here. Although sentimental work was core to their identities as nurses, the pressure to perform such tasks – as well as the delegation of these tasks by doctors – was negatively connoted. The complexity of the nursing role in performing sentimental work was reinforced by the frequent accounts of personal struggles to resolve a professional and/or personal desire to care with both the need for boundaries and the day-to-day stresses of managing time and clinical duties. As Strauss (1978) recognised, the order is reflective of a wider professional hierarchy. This was in all likelihood inflected by a historical gendered division of labour between nursing and medicine although this was not topicalised within the interviews.

The nurses' accounts illustrate their role and professional potency within the context of negotiations around the need for palliative care and in caring for the dying. In *doing* nursing more broadly, they are expected to establish intimacy and rapport with patients. In the context of futility, such forms of intimate work are clearly fundamental to the production of patient status and ensuring timely transitions to palliative and end-of-life care. The interviews reveal and reinforce nurses as having a defining role in the rules for interaction on the ward, and also in defining the patient's medical status (Strauss 1978). Yet, these nurses' accounts articulate an important division of labour between nursing and medicine in the context of futility and transitioning to the end of life, in part empowering nurses within the negotiated order of the hospital and in part relegating them to a particular form of engagement and *sentimental work* (Strauss et al. 1982). Nursing capital, at least in part, lies within the particular relations they maintain with patients and the day-to-day enactment of the 'nursing philosophy'. However, this comes at a price. It places considerable demands on nurses both in terms of balancing the performance of day-to-day, technical nursing, while doing caring and emotional work and maintaining the sentimental order within the ward (Strauss et al. 1982). It also positions them in a subordinate position whilst in some cases having superior insights into the life world of the dying patient and forms of suffering therein. Although a strength of nursing is clearly illustrated in these nurses' accounts, the competing and sometimes unrealistic demands being placed on nurses within this precarious, negotiated site of care offers considerable potential for suffering. Yet again we see how the politics and practices of professional distinction, and role differentiations, offer cost and benefit within a negotiated order in the nursing–medical relationship. This order of things in turn has clear influences over the management of futility and care for the dying.

# Chapter 7
# Dying, Healing and Survivorship

## Introduction

I have focused thus far on dying in the foreseeable future as something largely accepted by the individual, their families and the health professionals involved in their care and on the individuals who recognise, albeit to varying degrees, that the end of their life is approaching. This acceptance is certainly not the experience of all people who are considered from a biomedical perspective to be 'clinically terminal' or 'palliative' (Broom 2009a; Frank 2003; Hewitt et al. 2005; Kaiser 2008). A significant proportion of people who technically fit into those labels embark on practices of resistance and are unwilling to subscribe to biomedical prognostic predictions and they actively pursue and engage in practices of survivorship. This raises important questions: Are practices of resistance to 'terminal illness' inevitable in death-denying societies? Is resistance merely an artefact of denial or a more complex outcome of a reductive biomedical imposition of 'survival chances'? What do people *do* to resist terminality and what are the implications of such practices?

In this chapter I focus largely on the experiences of cancer patients, although the analysis extends well beyond this particular disease. Advanced cancer provides an important case study when thinking about resisting terminality and death and embarking on healing practices. One of the peculiarities of cancer is that the line between curable and incurable keeps moving. The steady production of new pharmacological agents, including new genetic therapies, means that what is possible for a person with cancer from a biomedical therapeutic perspective is constantly shifting. Major advances on the treatment of cancer (see Introduction for further discussion) have contributed to a cultural relation of hope, and have shaped the possibilities and expectations surrounding those who live with cancer. For those with cancer in long-term remission, increasingly cancer is becoming a chronic illness, including, for example, men with hormone responsive prostate cancer (Tritter and Calnan 2002; Phillips and Currow 2010). While fear of the 'cancer diagnosis' (Olson 2011; Stacey 1997) persists, therapeutic advances and community advocacy are heavily shaping the cultural perception of cancer. The proliferation of complementary and alternative medicine (CAM) in the context of cancer, has promoted ways of 'boosting' the immune system and the art of 'self-healing' through practitioner delivered and self-care practices. What this means is that being a 'terminal' cancer patient is an increasingly contested and problematic category (Sarenmalm et al. 2009; Frank 2001, 2003).

Therapy development and self-healing capacity – disparate but related socio-medical developments – have perpetuated a cultural discourse of *survival potential* and the necessity of the individual to resist 'losing the battle' with cancer and ultimately dying (Seale 2001, 2002; see also Sontag 1983). Many people with cancer thus embark on sustained practices of prognostic resistance and on a healing process, often in order to reclaim survivorship and individual agency (Broom 2009a). This, I argue, offers both possibility and problem for people living with advanced cancer.

What does any of this have to do with dying? The answer is quite evident to those working in palliative and end-of-life care. A significant proportion of people *never accept* they are dying. They embark on practices of healing and survivorship, as is shown in the data I present, often until their final days. Significantly, many people consider the act of prognosis (and biomedical survival chances) as a type of self-fulfilling prophecy. The imposition of a reductive population-based framework on an individual foments the loss of hope if the prognosis is internalised. This has profound implications for many people who live with cancer. The very categories of 'terminal' or 'incurable' are seen to produce what they speak of.

There is an increasing array of ontological and epistemological dilemmas in cancer and around 'terminality' that also involve significant practitioner disagreements (that is, between CAM and biomedicine) over who is dying and what possibilities exist for care and healing. In this chapter I focus on people's search for healing in advanced cancer and on accounts of reframing and/or rejecting 'being terminal'. I illustrate that while CAM practitioners and cancer 'gurus' may foster and facilitate biomedical prognostic resistance, such reframings may also pose new problems and reductive potential. Advanced cancer patients' engagement with CAM and cancer gurus, and how these are utilised to reconfigure and resist biomedical prognoses, is examined.

## Background

### *The Rise of 'Alternative Healing' in Advanced Cancer*

One of my reasons for this focus is because in recent years there has been a significant rise in the use of CAM practices and practitioners amongst advanced cancer patients (Bell 2010; Broom and Tovey 2007b, 2008; McClean 2005). There has also been a rise, particularly in Australia, of 'cancer gurus' who offer practitioner-directed and self healing to advanced cancer patients.

This has significantly shaped the cultural and social relations of hope and healing surrounding advanced cancer, as well as juxtaposed CAM approaches with medical oncology approaches (and other oncology specialties), invoking and provoking ideas about agency, individualism and even self-responsibility amongst patients (Bishop and Yardley 2004; McClean 2005). Many CAM modalities or practitioners and 'cancer gurus' have constructed *survivorship* as applying equally to advanced cancer patients as to people with biomedically 'curable' (or have been cured of) cancers. This has meant that people who are clinically 'dying' increasingly engage in survivorship/healing activities and processes of self-healing. This can involve radical lifestyle or ideological shifts (Bishop and Yardley 2004; McClean 2005), and the promotion of ideas about self-healing, positivity and the potency of the mind or self in surviving or overcoming cancer (De Raeve 1997; Gray and Doan 1990; Kissane 2009; Rittenberg 1995; see also Stacey 1997).

Drawing from individual accounts, I argue that the approaches taken by some CAM practitioners, and other cancer-specific healing models,[1] can be helpful but also can create a new normativity of *resisting dying* (see also Broom and Tovey 2008, Broom 2009b; Broom 2009a). These rather precarious spaces of cancer survivorship, often taking place well away from the gaze of biomedical oncology professionals, represent an important and under-researched site of care. Within these spaces people find techniques for encouraging survival and resisting dying, but also disciplinary and regressive ideas about the role of the individual at the end of life. In their practices of resistance we see cultural relations of virtue, control and individual responsibility (Broom 2009a, 2009b).

## *Surviving Terminality? Between Life and Death*

The stage in the cancer journey where one's disease is present and not requiring aggressive palliation, but is still 'uncontained', can be a highly liminal space (Little et al. 1998; Navona and Morag 2004). It can become a matter of waiting for disease to spread further (Sarenmalm et al. 2009). It is at this stage, betwixt and between survivor and dying, that CAM often presents as an attractive alternative (Broom 2009a). Many CAM practitioners provide forms of care that may fill the gap left when patients are offered no option from biomedicine other than palliative and end-of-life care. CAM practices and practitioners may also offer a sense of hope and a distinct 'survival trajectory' for advanced cancer patients

1 These tend to be systems of CAM that have developed from a charismatic or 'exceptional' individual who develops a system of care based on their 'successes'. Some examples include the Gawler foundation (see http://www.gawler.org and the Gerson institute http://www.gerson.org/).

(Broom and Tovey 2007b). In this sense, CAM practitioners are redefining the journey toward the end of life, particularly those phases where biomedicine may focus exclusively on pain management and quality of life rather than on longer term 'solutions'.

## *Subjectivity, Agency and Self-determination*

CAM practitioners may promote and enhance certain processes within the context of advanced cancer care including facilitating self-actualisation, empowerment and promoting an active role in the healing process (Barrett et al. 2003; Broom and Tovey 2007b). Research illustrates that CAM practitioners may be influential in the reinsertion of subjectivity into therapeutic processes, promote self-healing and hope, and facilitate a sense of agency and individual autonomy (e.g. Barrett et al. 2003; Bishop and Yardley 2004; Broom and Tovey 2007b; Broom 2009b). This is not artificially juxtaposing CAM with biomedical (advanced) cancer care. Many of the aspects of CAM care are evident in biomedical oncological settings and there are some CAM practices that involve little direct or even indirect engagement with ideas about personhood, self-care, holism or subjectivity (medical acupuncture or aromatherapy massage are good examples). While complex and differentiated across professions and between practitioners, CAM users' accounts illustrate some of the broader differences in emphasis between CAM and biomedicine. A central pillar of and consistency between many CAM approaches to cancer is ontological in character (Broom 2009c); ideas about the reconstruction of reality and the power of the mind in living with and overcoming cancer. Often involving mindfulness techniques or other self-directed forms of self-care, these models of 'work on the self' as 'work on disease' depart significantly from biomedical approaches to cancer and palliative care.

These are not novel ideas and there is an established literature (some positive, some negative) on the 'reconstruction of reality' in the context of advanced cancer (De Raeve 1997; Gray and Doan 1990; Rittenberg 1995). However, an ontology of 'work on the self' that 'works on advanced cancer' is becoming increasingly evident in many CAM practices and this framing of disease (and the person) has both liberating and coercive potential. The coercive aspect, often drawn from neo-Buddhist ideas about *wellbeing* and *presence*, transforms survival into a matter of peaceful self-determination, at least in part (Broom and Tovey 2008; Broom 2009a, 2009c). The rather contradictory requirements of 'being strong' and 'being at peace' situate advanced cancer experiences as reflective of personal virtue, charismatic presence and thus self-worth, components that I characterise here as a moral framing of alternative healing (see also Frank 1997;

and Booth 1994 on moral economy). The key questions that emerge are who is this practice for and to what ends?

## *Virtue, Obligation and the Moral Economy of Survivorship*

The virtues of 'the good fight' have been deconstructed previously (e.g. Gray and Doan 1990; Frank 1997; Hart, Sainsbury and Short 1998; Seale 2001) and critique of the moral framing of illness and dying is well developed in the academic literature (Chattoo and Ahmad 2008; Meyer 1995; Mohammed and Peter 2009). In the context of CAM and advanced cancer, such moralities are often embedded in the cultural need to enact 'timely deaths' (Booth 1994) manifest in interpersonal forms of reciprocity and mutual obligation that encourage advanced cancer sufferers to 'rise to the occasion' (Frank 1997). These cultural practices intermingle with existing and emerging techniques of self-management and self-actualisation (Bolletino 2001). Whereas biomedical cancer care is often about 'enduring' chemotherapy or other biomedical externally-imposed toxicities, in the context of CAM it is often about the *virtue*s of acceptance and self-awareness. Such models of survivorship are very beneficial for some people. In advanced cancer and those nearing the end of life there is potential for CAM practitioners (and more extreme 'cancer gurus') to be complicit in the production of reductive survivorship discourses (Broom 2009a). These ideas position survivorship, even in the face of end stage disease, as a *moral imperative* through an ontology of mind–body–spirit connectivity (Bolletino 2001). Through virtue and control of the self (fear, doubt, anxiety), we can actively reconstruct our realities and bodies as a pathway to moving beyond advanced cancer.

I argue that such discourses and technologies of care at the end of life may be producing a new type of self-governance and repressive possibilities that morally bind its subjects to 'fight on'. The extreme focus on agency and self-determination ultimately positions CAM practices and 'cancer gurus' as subject–reductive rather than object–reductive (the latter being a common criticism of biomedicine). These ideas often fit neatly into the life worlds of stakeholders surrounding the patient (family, partners, carers) who may hope for a heroic (Gray and Doan 1990) and timely (Parry 1994) death. Herein lie the new forms and techniques of governance of 'the good fight' beyond the realm of biomedicine. And there is complicity from within this increasingly prominent group of CAM practitioners in the moral framing of living with and dying of cancer. When we examine the experiences of advanced cancer patients themselves we see the tensions around, and trouble with, self-help and self-care. I draw on data from a British study and an Australian study of advanced cancer patients to illustrate and provide insight into these issues.

## Into the Field

### *The Control–Responsibility Dialectic*

In 2007–2008 I studied Australian (Brisbane-based) highly active CAM users who were living with advanced cancer, the majority of whom were clinically in line for 'palliative and supportive care only'. In clinical terms that they were 'terminal' or 'incurable'. My recruitment strategy was designed to target those advanced cancer patients using CAMs more intensively rather than occasional users, thereby providing in-depth insight into the CAM life-world in the context of advanced cancer. I recruited from medical oncology wards in Brisbane, Australia, to retain some degree of spread of people living with advanced cancer. The majority were using a combination of CAM practices, including but not limited to ingested practices (for example, dietary regimens), practitioner healing (for example, energy, spiritual) and alternative self-care (for example, yoga, meditation, mindfulness). The majority were also receiving some form of biomedical care and often their CAM activities were unknown to their oncologist or palliative care physician. I was interested in the role of more active or radical CAM engagement particularly the desire to embark on a healing process and even cure in the context of terminality.

The interviews were revealing in terms of the radical role CAM practices and practitioners played in the lives of patients and the influence on their views of living with cancer. Their *early interview talk* reflected the potency of self-responsibility and CAM healing practices that encouraged human agency. I start with these initial reflections:

> *Participant* (female): The bottom line is I think you have to have some control in all of this … The only thing you have control about, are things that you can put into your body that are easily accessible.

Another participant comments:

> *Participant* (female): … I eat apricot kernels like they're going out of fashion … I've become very peaceful about it all really. But I do believe that you can control areas of the body and that they [CAMs] can help to shrink the cancer away and suppress it too I suppose.

Another participant comments:

> *Participant* (female): To this day I still meditate every morning – just 6 to 7. I don't sit up, hey, I've got breast cancer; I can do this lying down. I'm not hard on

> myself any more and I had found all of that ... I really needed to bring myself to a place of relaxation ... to self-heal.

It is worth noting that the majority of the participants in this particular study had been given months or perhaps a year to live. Initially in the interviews, their CAM-derived healing pathways were presented as hugely positive in relation to the limited biomedical options available. The hope inspired by CAM practitioners and practices around 'healing' was talked about with statements such as 'this is the only thing keeping me going' and 'the only thing positive about this whole thing'. However, later in the interviews, a different set of accounts emerged around self-healing discourse and the omnipresent pressure to think positive and be vigilant:

> *Participant* (female): I tend not to get desperate about things. I've gotta think positive and ... [pauses and thinks for a while] I think that people who *have* to think positive, that deep down they're not. The fact that they've *gotta* force themselves to be positive, means that consciously they're being positive but subconsciously ... it just drips away.

Another participant comments:

> *Participant* (female): Um ... to be honest in a lot of cases alternative medicine seems too hard. To, for instance, change diet drastically, um yeah, it's hard with food ... the thought of eating horrible food really puts me off and I don't think I could go vegetarian ... to maintain the self-discipline and be good all the time.

Another participant comments:

> *Participant* (female): For me, I suppose positivity allows me to help myself. So helping myself is a cure for cancer, that's how I receive it. Because I know that if you're not positive, you can feel it, you know. It's acidic in your belly and everything. So that's how I think ... take the negativity out of your body ... it's very hard. It's a challenge every day because there are times I cry. No one sees it, but I cry, you know? I cry because what more can I do? It's a challenge every day ... You have to just be vigilant.

The potentially restrictive nature of continued positivity and consciousness-based self-healing, often espoused by many self-help gurus and CAM practitioners, emerged as a prominent theme in the interviews. While each participant agreed with the importance of taking a broadly positive approach – *and such ideas were viewed as central to their survival* – hyperpositivity and illusory forms of 'self-healing' were seen as counterproductive and as concealing a grieving process or underlying fear of terminality and dying. Performing positivity, as several interviewees stated, was viewed as relatively appealing at one level as it feeds into the needs of those around you (family and friends). The sense of potency over an otherwise incurable disease was initially very attractive to the patient and carer or family. However, as disease progresses and positivity is tested, the need to 'be happy' and 'be positive' acts as a disciplinary mechanism, rather than a therapeutic device. Surviving and *resisting dying* becomes about personal *virtue* and an act of *moral obligation* rather than necessarily a desirable state. Indeed, the interviewees often talked about the initial therapeutic potential of radical alternative healing models followed by reflection on the dark underbelly of alternative cancer self-help programs and practices. The desire to 'put on a brave face' to CAM practitioners and family and friends resulted in ongoing repression of feelings of hopelessness and self-doubt. Examination of the temporal dimensions of CAM engagement provides an even more vivid illustration of such processes.

### *Temporality and Ontological Change*

While an interview-based 'snapshot' understanding of healing and survivorship illustrates a person's experience at a particular time point, in order to tease out the dynamics of healing over time it is useful to engage in other forms of data collection. A temporal analysis can be useful as people with advanced cancer may start off with, or even perform, positivity in their interview-based accounts of living with advanced cancer, but do their experiences change over time? In the qualitative interview there are performative aspects of the researcher–researched relationship; there is a desire to be positive and this can shape accounts of illness and care. I had the first opportunity in 2005–06 to undertake a diary-based study with advanced cancer patients who were receiving care from the British National Health Service. Subsequently, I have undertaken several other diary-based studies given the success of the initial study (see Broom et al. 2014b; Broom et al. 2014c). I draw on the first diary study in particular here.

In this British study I asked eight people living with advanced cancer, who I had interviewed previously, to complete a one month diary of their CAM use, self-healing practices and living with cancer. Each participant was a very active CAM user when given the diary. I interviewed each participant before and after they completed the diary. The idea was to get a sense of CAM engagement and survivorship as *everyday activities*, with ups and downs. While all eight represented CAM practices and practitioners in a very positive light in the initial interview (as highly motivational, critical to their survivorship and as giving them hope) it was evident in the diaries that such perceptions did not necessarily persist over time. Their diaries reveal, to an even greater extent than the interview data presented in the previous section, a new normativity of alternative self-healing in the context of advanced cancer. In the following diary excerpts we see the day-to-day struggle of attempting to keep up enthusiasm for a CAM self-healing regimen for advanced cancer and the crucial role encounters with biomedical and CAM clinicians play in driving or delimiting the ability of patients to maintain focus and enthusiasm.

*Participant* (male):

Day 1: [The participant lists a substantial dietary and supplement regimen costing over £2000 a month including daily caffeine enemas] Although it seems like a lot to be taking it is fairly easy to regulate and really gives me the feeling like I am actively doing something every day. In addition to the pills I also try to do a coffee enema every day … I feel well in myself and have had neither positive nor negative thoughts …

Day 2: I woke up feeling depressed but after I went round to a friend's house and had a nice chat I felt much better. Then I received a phone call from [CAM practitioner] who told me he could see a definite improvement in my lymph. I went to bed feeling very positive.

Day 9: I am having a CT scan on the seventeenth of this month. I know that the results will look worse than my first CT scan. The doctors will stress upon me how important it is to have chemo. I do not want to hear how important it is to have chemo. I do not want to hear that as it will cast doubt and fear into my mind and it is important to stay positive … What a crazy world we try to live in [sic].

Day 17: A CT scan at the hospital today. Spoke to the nurse who was very supportive of my alternative approach. That's the kind of attitude I want from the doctors – not denouncing the unknown … At the end of Yoga today I asked the instructor if there were any exercises I could do that stimulated lymph flow. He told me some. I told him why I wanted to do this and cried. When I got home I cried again, like when I first found the lump and had to tell people I cried. It was nice to let go of some emotion.

*Diary entries missing for a couple of days …*

Day 24: Chatted with [my friend] today. I told [my friend] I found it difficult to keep motivated as I feel so well. Sometimes I have to remind myself that I'm ill, sometimes I slack off a bit for a few days, don't do enemas, don't lymphasise etc … However, I do always take my supplements.

A particular emphasis in the above diary entries, and those of the other eight participants, was the flux in motivation for CAM over time; a perhaps self-evident but also often understated aspect of CAM utilisation in advanced cancer care. Ironically, sometimes the hardest moments in terms of being *self-disciplined* in maintaining a particular therapeutic approach were when the participants felt well and happy with their lives. There seemed to be an underlying tension between the need to 'heal oneself' through CAM, whilst minimising how much time and 'headspace' it demanded. The day-to-day enactment of CAM was riddled with a personal struggle over not wanting to 'miss the good moments' (as a result of focusing too much on self-healing) but needing to be disciplined (remembering that 'healing' takes self-discipline). Certainly, in each of the diaries an element of self-disciplining was evident; an undertone that is likely linked to wider discourses of the self within therapeutic culture (Rose 1999). These patients articulated in their dairies the need to 'think differently' about cancer, to seek 'self-healing' and minimise 'negativity'. Moreover, as shown in another participant's diary entries below, carers and family members' encouragement was critical within the wider problematic of heroic survivorship and CAM engagement.

> *Participant* (female):
>
> Day 2: … I cannot talk to my family, it gets too emotional, they always say, "you are strong, you will beat it" …
>
> Day 3: I do wish that some friends would discuss my illness but because I always try to put on a good front, I must give the impression I don't want to discuss it.

These participants' diaries, along with the interview data in the previous section and other studies, illustrate that while CAM-derived techniques of self-determination and self-healing can be useful at certain points, they also created a form of governance of the self, a process whereby patients felt guilty if they 'slept in', 'missed an enema' or 'had negative thoughts'. Motivation for healing necessarily involves retaining a sense of pathology or 'unwellness' – an interesting paradox. This has important implications for how we think about CAM, survivorship and 'terminal illness' sociologically. As a general rule, CAM practitioners do not focus on the terminality of disease or indeed on biomedically-conceived survival chances. Rather, there remains a focus on healing, self-actualisation or cleansing the body. At least for these patients, the day-to-day act of 'doing CAM' necessarily involved remembering the root causes of one's need for healing (and thus the presence of advanced disease). This was accompanied by the sense that, healing would only come through resolution (and comfort) with one's body, one's 'self' and *one's disease*. Such an outcome, however, could only be achieved through taking a disciplined approach to self-healing and fully accepting an alternative conception of health, disease and the self. The conflict of motivation coming from a need to 'feel well' and wellness as limiting motivation ('I just want to enjoy the time I have left') was an important theme in these diaries.

### *Dying to Survive? The Toxic Combination of Futility and Virtue in Advanced Cancer*

A strength of the temporal nature of this study of British advanced cancer patients was its ability to capture key moments of transition in cancer patients' engagement with CAM and self-healing practices. Although I gave them a diary for only one month, even during this short period changes were evident in several of their approaches to CAM. For example, one participant went through a transition from active self-healing and following a rigorous CAM regime to in-patient end-of-life care. The following diary excerpt from his last few weeks of life provides an illustration of how self-help and self-healing practices can be problematic near death. For this particular patient, the diary recorded his last month of life. Previously, he had pursued a rigorous dietary regimen called the Gerson diet, and had attended (costly) weekend meetings with his wife in CAM/healing centres in cities other than where he lived. When he was first interviewed for this study, he and his wife were ardent supporters of the Gerson diet, spending hours a day preparing food and juicing in order to detoxify the body according to this treatment program (nine kilograms of crushed fruit and vegetables a day, with hourly glasses of juice, in combination with 3–4 coffee enemas). Both in their 80s, this program was very strenuous and was a large commitment. The diary begins at a time when he was becoming weaker yet still aiming for long-term survival, with friends and clinicians concerned that the CAM treatments were too much. What follows is an emotional and difficult movement away from a rigorous diet, to a process of acceptance of death and an acknowledgement of finality.

> *Participant* (male):
>
> Day 9: Attended [CAM practitioners] consulting room … We learned more about the Gerson [diet] There are three doctors in the UK who have received Gerson training and who claim Gerson credentials but they have their own interpretation. For me this is confusing and part of medical politics and ego. He [CAM practitioner] talked quite knowingly about the treatment but when I asked him to point out the injection site [for the treatment] on my buttocks he was not certain … He suggested I take two or three juices a day plus a coffee enema until we geared up for the full treatment.

> Day 13: I slept indifferently despite the visualisation described on the Bristol tape of a healing blue light falling on me. Probably my visualisation needs to be improved since I do not produce a clear mental picture but rather a vague adumbrated picture …
>
> Day 14: Visited [doctor's name] who is very sympathetic and warns me not to be so ardent in self denial but to listen to my body's requirements.
>
> Day 15: [6am] Started to prepare carrots and apples for the day's juicing … I time the procedure to be about three hours
>
> Day 20: [Support group leader] came to see me after a session. I asked her why they were so against me using the Gerson Therapy. She explained that it is a very demanding and time consuming therapy and the clinic did not consider it wise at our age … This was a very valid point. I think that whilst I have made a critical change it will be best all round [to change to something else] and give us a quality of life together that Gerson could ruin.
>
> Day 22: We have changed course to a less severe therapy therefore more suited to our age.
>
> *Admitted to hospital due to infection.*
>
> Day 23: I'm awake at 4 am. I have resolve to attempt to modify my diet and exercise more as a self-help therapy. Life is difficult though now I'm on steroids and I don't know how to balance diet, rest, exercise … I am informed that a special bed will be delivered sometime tonight to relieve my sores. I have been thinking of sitting in the chair all night with a blanket around me.
>
> *The above notes are the last Alan wrote in this diary. Four weeks later he died at 7:30 am. His wife delivered the diary and gave a follow-up interview.*

The experience, and indeed difficulties, of utilising CAM approaches in the context of advanced disease is vividly shown in this participant's last few weeks before he died and is also borne out in the other diaries and subsequent studies (see Broom 2009a, 2009b). When I first interviewed the above participant he was mobile, feeling healthy and actively pursuing a self-healing and long-term survivorship/curative strategy. The rigorous diet and mindfulness regimen was no longer tenable as his condition worsened and he was then hospitalised. His support networks and family were hugely concerned about such a rigorous diet and eventually he acknowledged this too. The example clearly raises the issue of just how tenable and durable certain CAM and self-healing models are, and their disciplinary potential. Ideologies espousing individual healing put very specific demands on patients with advanced cancer who are terminally ill, producing an overwhelming guilt around 'not being disciplined enough' or 'not keeping positive'. Such observations indicate the role of CAM practices and practitioners and contemporary 'cancer gurus' in the perpetuation of notions of *duty* and *virtue* in cancer survivorship, and how they may morally bind people's journeys through normative (and unrealistic) nations of 'acceptance', 'peacefulness' and 'transcendence'. Both the above studies illustrate that such 'virtuous practices' are ultimately relational in character, and are situated within cultural ideas about obligation and reciprocity within the context of family/ carer dynamics.

## Discussion

My aim in this chapter has been to elaborate further the complexity of dying as a *social process* – and one that is heavily inflected by emerging social movements including those of CAM and self-care. CAM practices and practitioners are increasingly playing important roles in advanced cancer and in end-of-life care (for example, mindfulness, reiki, acupuncture, massage). CAM practices and practitioners have important roles, however, there is a more aggressive and reductive aspect of contemporary healing in the context of advanced cancer promoted by *some* CAM practitioners. This presents a new array of dilemmas on those considered 'terminal' as people seek to reconcile competing ideas about survival chances. Moreover, it shapes their pathways to the end of life.

As I suggested above, many people simply do not accept they are 'terminal' or indeed dying. From a sociological perspective, what is important is the individual's experience, not historical survival data. But what is interesting is what people *do* within these spaces of resistance and how they seek to reclaim control and a sense of agency within the disease process and whether, for them, they achieve their aims. I have examined a particular subset of advanced cancer patients; those specifically interested in resisting biomedical notions of futility through utilising CAM practices and practitioners. And I have critically explored this space, seeking to understand both the potential *and* problematic in regards to alternative self-healing in advanced cancer. I would argue that sociologists have illustrated a lack of willingness to explore the more disciplinary or controlling aspects of alternative health practices and practitioners, despite much protest from biomedicine, who are often perceived to be too 'against CAM' to maintain credible positions. Here, I have aimed to provide a more balanced view of survival practices in the context of advanced 'incurable' cancer, practices of resistance to terminality and the role of CAM therein.

Disciplinary devices and pathological ontologies operate across the health and medical professions and practices (see Bell 2010; and Good et al. 1990). Indeed, notions of 'survival-through-character', 'health-through-discipline', and 'survivorship-as-individual-heroism' have too often been visible in mainstream oncology settings and in broader public health initiatives. Coercive and totalising narratives of survival exist well beyond CAM. However, the ways in which some CAM practitioners are 'doing' disciplinarity in the context of advanced cancer and 'terminal illness' is quite unique and requires specific attention.

There is a 'transformation of care' occurring in advanced 'terminal' cancer and CAM techniques and discourses are playing a central role for many patients. It is rather ironic that despite CAM emerging as a pertinent and timely critique of biomedical mastery over bodies and health, CAM-derived ideas about 'wellbeing', 'self-help' and 'self-responsibility' also represent new sites of governance of the self, the body and of health (cf. Rose 1999). There is a normative and coercive potential to self-help and self-healing discourse and practice. Just as biomedicine has received ongoing critique for its role in reductive models of health and illness, there is a real need for an examination of the role of CAM practices and practitioners' in problematising advanced cancer and cancer survivorship experiences, and in shaping the contemporary experience of dying, including capacity and willingness to accept or embrace the end of life.

Specifically, there is a need for consideration as to how new conceptions of disease and selfhood may actually facilitate a governing of the subject. Rose's (1999) work on governmentality and therapeutic culture more broadly may be useful. He suggests that in the second half of the twentieth century 'the very idea of health was reconfigured [to] encode an optimisation of one's corporeality to embrace a kind of overall well-being'. This, he argues, has been amplified by self-help movements, therapeutic culture and alternative therapeutics which engender a 'working on the self' (Rose 2001) as one element of good citizenship. Individuals are thus colonised by discursive models of selfhood and agency that are not, strictly speaking, their own (Murray 2007). The flip side of so-called subjectification and individualised conceptions of the self (in tandem with wider discourses and self-help and wellbeing) may actually constrain the subject (Rose 1999), creating dilemmas between self-actualisation and empowerment and self-responsibility and disciplinary effects (Foucault 1988; see also Armstrong 2007).

Another important emphasis has been on how cancer survivorship is intimately intertwined with the politics of virtue, obligation and reciprocity (Broom and Cavenagh 2010), that is, how CAM models may interplay with a broader cultural desire to ensure a 'timely death' (Parry 1982, 1994) – a process that can emerge from an interactional morality based on struggle as virtue. Further work is needed to document how people who are 'terminal' and perhaps 'dying' negotiate these cultural scripts and personal meanings. It is worth considering whether CAM models of care are complicit in a new moral framing of advanced cancer survivorship (see also Chattoo and Ahmad 2008) and that such *moralities of survivorship* produce interpersonal dilemmas about a responsibility to live as long as one can, a responsibility to be at 'peace', and a responsibility to reconstruct one's bodily and emotional reality.

Every model of care contains reductive components and the ideas of self-actualisation, self-healing and self-responsibility are not prima facie bad. In fact, there are some very important aspects of CAM that must be considered alongside its potential for harm or negative effects. For many in palliative and end-of-life care contexts, CAM practices and practitioners provide vital support for physiological, psychological and spiritual needs. For example, the focus on achieving wellbeing as opposed to 'cure', 'more time' or 'long-term remission', may be quite empowering for some advanced cancer patients and their families. In taking this emphasis, CAM approaches and practitioners may be more attuned to the embodied and intuitive experiences of having (and coping with) advanced cancer. Indeed, CAM practices and practitioners may better encapsulate notions of *authenticity* (of being true to one's own spirit or being, regardless of external structures or models), of *recognition* (the external acknowledgement of the validity of subjective experience) and of *individual agency* (the individual as central and powerful in the healing process) (see Sointu 2006a, 2006b, 2006c). I have documented in some depth elsewhere the highly positive features of many CAM practices for cancer patients, including promoting a greater sense of agency and power in their therapeutic trajectories (see Broom 2009a, 2009b, 2009c).

However, the assumption of agency and individuation (something that conceptually has been engendered in much sociology in this area) should be checked through an exploration of various disciplinary devices, techniques and methods of imposing self-governance; processes that may indeed be problematic for those individuals attempting to cope with a life limited, and the transition to the end of their life. The assumption of agency and individuation also should be balanced by an exploration of the transformation of a discrete physical disease into a problem involving all areas of a person's life – a process described by Sered and Agigian (2008) as 'holistic sickening' – and the implications for patient journeys through care/illness and toward the end of life.

# Chapter 8
# Gender and the Moralities of Dying

## Introduction

Dying is a morally and politically laden social process that is deeply embedded in gendered social relations (e.g. Broom 2012b), as well as in other important social relations including class, age and ethnicity (e.g. Howarth 2007c). Just as gender plays a strong role on mediating other human experiences (Broom and Tovey 2009), so too gender mediates experiences near death and the dying process (Field, Hockey and Small 1997). While it has been acknowledged that experiences of dying are strongly determined by identity issues (Hallam, Hockey and Howarth 1999), this remains an under-researched area of inquiry (Broom 2012b). While I certainly do not seek to engage on all aspects of gender dynamics and dying in this chapter, I do seek to begin a discussion around gender identities at the end of life, with a focus on masculinities and relations of care in particular. I posit that dying is surrounding by a particular set of (evolving) gendered moral scripts, and that these require significant investigation to understand and potentially improve experiences near death.

While there has been some work done on gender as manifest within the dying process (for example, Broom 2012b; Field, Hockey and Small 1997), the emphasis of palliative and end-of-life care research more broadly has tended to be on the physiological and psychological management of pain and suffering. This has meant limited exploration of the challenges to gender identities and roles in palliative and end-of-life care settings, including evolving and gendered moral codes (Kellehear 2008; Thomas, Morris and Harman 2002; McPherson, Wilson and Murray 2007). In combination with other facets of individual biographies, gender identities mediate patient and carer preferences, interactions with clinical staff and even intervention requests at the end of life (Broom 2012b; Kellehear 2008; Kirsi, Hervonen and Jylha 2004; Lawton 2000; McPherson, Wilson and Murray 2007; Parsons 1997).

Through an exploration of key issues related to morality, dignity and 'the good death', in this chapter I examine some important intersections of gender and dying. Rather than seeking to develop a 'sex role' understanding of dying, I present a constructivist-driven exploration of how contemporary gender scripts and forms of identity interplay (differentially) with the dying process for different individuals. Despite several key sociological studies and texts emerging over the last few decades (e.g. Glaser and Strauss 1965, 1968; Kellehear 1990; Kubler-Ross 1969; Lawton 2000; Prior 1989; Seale 1998a), there has been a paucity of work on how hospice and palliative care experiences may vary according to biographies. This chapter represents the beginning of a wider discussion of some of the evolving gendered dimensions of dying, grounded in the stories and experiences of hospice patients and families themselves.

## Background

### *Debating the 'Good Death'*

In thinking about gender and dying it is first worth revisiting the wider moral and political economy of dying, some of which I touched on in the Introduction and in previous chapters. Within the sociology of death and dying there has been regular debate over the politics and ideological purposes of ideas about 'the good death' (Gott et al. 2008; Hart, Sainsbury and Short 1998; see also Seale 1998a). On the one hand, the notion of 'the good death' has been deployed within the hospice movement to signify death with dignity, peace and comfort (Kubler-Ross 1969). On the other hand, 'the good death' has been critiqued as a form of social control (McNamara, Waddell and Colvin 1994, 1995) and as potentially marginalising divergent forms and experiences of dying (Hart, Sainsbury and Short 1998). These concerns are enhanced within a context of a growing recognition that the capacity to 'die well', within any given normative framework, may be different between different groups of individuals (Howarth 2007c). Yet, contemporary palliative and hospice care is still largely underpinned by particular models of 'dying well'. The 'revivalist' good death, for example, described by Clark (2002: 907), reflects an agenda within palliative care that a 'good death' should feature such things as: 'being pain free', 'acceptance', 'closure', 'awareness' and 'individuality' among other things (see also Seale 1998b). While such components are not prima facie problematic, their normative and prescriptive potential is worth considering – as I have in previous chapters – how gender may inflect engagement with such moralities of dying. Models of 'dying well' have tended to be driven by academic and clinical perspectives, with little research evidence available on what patients themselves believe to be 'a good death' (see for an exception Gott et al. 2008; also Kendall et al. 2007).

The research available suggests patients' views of 'a good death' may conflict with the values upon which palliative care is predicated (Gott et al. 2008). In their study Gott et al. (2008) found that older people's views of 'a good death' often conflict with the 'revivalist' model, with their participants not desiring open awareness of death, acknowledgement of the imminence of dying, or not supporting the concepts of autonomy and individuality (Gott et al. 2008). I was interested in exploring hospice patients' views of different forms of death and dying ('good', 'bad' or otherwise) and how these reflections would be shaped by their own biographies including their gender identities? In other areas of health and illness patient experiences have been shown to be greatly influenced by gender, ethnicity and class (Hallam, Hockey and Howarth 1999; Howarth 2007c), yet little work has been done on hospice patients' perspectives. This paucity of research is particularly the case for the study of masculinities and dying.

### *The 'Good Death' as Gendered*

Howarth (2007c) argues that there has been a privileging of middle-class 'verbalised' versus working-class 'stoical' forms of dying and caring in the academic literature. Similarly, the influence of masculine identities within the dying process has not been given significant attention. Lawton (2000) touched on the interplay of hospice care and gender identity, suggesting a potential 'degenderisation' of hospice patients through loss of capacity to 'do gender' (particularly though their sexual contact). Such an analysis, from my perspective, tends toward a binary conception of gender (gender identity as either maintained or lost) and, furthermore, may overstate the centrality of sexuality in the performativity of gender at the end of life (see Lawton 2000: 168). I argue for a wider view of the interplay of masculinity and dying that extends to the potential loss of cultural and interpersonal roles (Broom and Tovey 2008). This is situated within an understanding that there has been a tendency within the social sciences to interpret end-of-life experiences as largely undifferentiated in their bodily and emotional impact (Howarth 2007c). I argue that a more nuanced conception of dying is necessary, and exploring the role of contemporary masculinities is an important starting point (Emslie et al. 2009; Parsons 1997). This necessarily includes, I would suggest, reflection on the experiences of being cared for.

### *Gendering Dying and Caring*

The gendered politics of caring has been well documented in the sociological literature (for example, Field et al. 1993; James 1989; Thomas, Morris and Harman 2002), and feminist researchers have emphasised the negative consequences of informal caring for women (for example, Thomas 1993). Research on caring has traditionally examined the hidden and feminine character of this work (Emslie et al. 2009; Exley and Letherby 2001), whereas the experiences of men and those people who men care for have been given relatively little attention (see Emslie et al. 2009; Kirsi et al. 2004; Parsons 1997; also Crocker 2002; Karp and Tanarugsachock 2000). In the context of hospice and palliative care, research has indicated that carers might underplay their own needs while trying to represent the voice of the person needing care (Grande, Todd and Barclays 1997). And taking a more theoretical bent, caring for the dying has been examined as moral practice; as a site of inter-subjectivity involving the reconstitution of the 'competent social agent' (Chattoo and Ahmad 2008). Moral practice as articulated in previous chapters, in this context, denotes ideas about how people should treat others and be treated by them, including, as Sayer (2005) posits, matters of justice and fairness and relations of recognition, care and friendship. Yet, little is known about how notions of responsibility, gift and reciprocity operate from the dying person's perspective and how this plays out in terms of gendered relations. There has been sporadic research in selected out-patient palliative care settings which has illustrated the gendered character of the carer–cared-for dynamic, including forms of intense emotional labour and the desire to maintain gender roles or dynamics (for example Emslie et al. 2009; Exley and Letherby 2001).

## Into the Field

### *What is a 'Good Death'?*

In this chapter I draw on the aforementioned qualitative study of an in-patient hospice patient in NSW, Australia (see previous chapters for details.As discussed above, what constitutes 'a good death' has been the source of much debate in the biomedical and social science literature and I wanted to examine the framing of different forms of death and dying in conversation with hospice in-patients themselves. While I do not present the following accounts as in any way definitive in terms of wider patient preferences, they provide some important reflections for understanding dying phenomenologically. There emerged a diverse set of preferences in and around death and dying, with a complex array of factors mediating these, including carer needs and perceptions of burden:

> *Participant* (female): I think you've got to fight for your life. I think we all do every day, don't we? We step out in front of a car, fine. You know? But we can back off from the car, we don't have to step in front of it, that's our prerogative, that's our life.

Another respondent comments:

> *Interviewer*: For you, what is a good death?
>
> *Participant* (female): I'm not even sure if I know that [pauses]. I do know that I'd like there to just be an ongoing sense of peace, and no traumas in my life, no family dramas … for as long as I can I will stay alive and do something, I'm not going to just lie here in this bed until the day I die, I've got other things I'd like to do.

Another respondent comments:

> *Interviewer*: … What is a good death?
>
> *Participant* (male): We can't run away from it, so we might as well face it, be as fully prepared for it as we can, sort of thing …. It's just sort of, letting you go with a bit of dignity, a bit of decorum, and ah, just seeing you through it as comfortably as possible … I mean if they're [your family] going to have to see you die, which they are, they'd much prefer to see you lying there, nice and comfortable, and all zonked out and can't talk to them, sort of thing. Rather than to be spewin' or, you know, being a big mess, running around struggling for breath.

Another respondent comments:

> *Participant* (male): I know [wife's name] wants me to hang around as long as I can. Um, no, I've got no intentions of giving up, I've got every intention of fighting it for as long as I can. Um, you're fighting a losing battle, but what the hell, you've got to be in it! … My own preference, as I said, would've been to have a sudden death. But, you don't get your preference, you don't get a choice. You get whatever cards were dealt.

Another respondent comments:

> *Participant* (male): [She] wouldn't want me to give up. For her, I'll hang on, you know?

The participants' accounts of death and dying were hugely varied and contained a mix of struggle talk and the desire for 'an end'. As shown in the above excerpts, and in several of the other interviews, doing the good death was often articulated as 'not giving up' and 'fighting for your life. There was often an emphasis placed on achieving peace and calmness in the final moments, and a death that was 'not messy' for relatives. It was interesting to note that almost unanimously the participants' talk of the 'good death' engendered the idea that one should and can 'rise to the occasion' (Frank 1997: 134; see also May 1991). This moral framing of dying permeated our discussions within the interviews. It was not that the participants simply accepted externally prescribed ideas about how to die and focused on achieving 'the good death', rather, that ideas (personal and cultural) about 'good deaths' were articulated, reconfigured *and* contested within the interviews, with oscillation evident between embracing and resisting different 'expectations' in and around death and dying. The 'good death' emerged as a site of considerable personal and interpersonal tension whereby the needs and desires of the dying person, interplayed with those of the carers, family and hospice staff.

As Sayer reflects (2005), morality is necessarily about relations to others; about how people should treat one another in ways conducive to mutual wellbeing. The interviews reflected interpersonal struggle over how to manage such relations while also maintaining a sense of an authentic self. I should emphasise that the idea of dying as moral practice does not reduce 'fighting' and 'struggling' talk to mere cultural pressure or mutual obligation. Indeed, this would deny these participants' agency and recognition of the legitimate desire to ascribe meaning to the end of life. As Chattoo and Ahmad (2008) argue, externally referential action does not necessarily denote an absence of agency. In fact, drawing on Tronto (1993) they argue that morality is a form of agency, arguing for a view of moral practice in the caring–dying relationship as 'relational autonomy'. Such arguments, as Sayer (2005: 952) notes, position forms of moral practice as containing both normative and liberative elements; moral beliefs sometimes endorse inequalities and relations of deference and condescension, but they also embody notions of fairness and relations of recognition, care and friendship.

The importance and centrality of 'dying well' as moral and ethical practice was evident in the participants' accounts, despite the level of emotional labour required. This included implicit and explicit talk of managing their own feelings (for example, fear, exhaustion and frustration) and those of their carers. Yet, underlying their accounts of emotional labour, were stories of desirable deaths (see also Payne, Langley-Evans and Hillier 1996) and resistance to the moral practice of 'rising to the occasion'. Without wanting to be seen as reneging on their willingness to do 'a slow death', there was an idealised vision of 'how others go':

> *Participant* (male): Yeah, I mean, right now, if I had my choices, if you could pick the way to go, I would choose to go the way my grandfather did, which was coming out of the paddock to have breakfast, grabbed his little grandson, put him on his knee, said to grandma that he was ready for his porridge, and he put his brown sugar on his porridge, and his home made butter, and was stirring it all in there, and dropped dead of a heart attack. Now that's the way to go if you've got a choice.

Another respondent comments:

> *Participant* (male): A good death? Quick. My wife had a beautiful death. I think now, although not at the time when she died.

Another respondent comments:

> *Participant* (male): Yeah. Getting it over and done with, and ah, have my funeral and ah, my wife suffer very little if possible. I know it will be a trying time for her. But, you see, there's no light bulb to switch off, you just, you've gotta lie here until nature takes its course. Maybe I get pneumonia, or maybe I get blood clots, I don't know, but I want it over with. I don't want to have this kind of life.

The desire to hasten death in advanced cancer patients in not a new observation (see Kelly et al. 2002), but the interviews revealed more than merely a desire to 'end it' quickly. What the interviews illustrated was the contradictory feelings and desires at the end of life that often go unexpressed due to a range of interpersonal pressures and cultural expectations. The moral practice of embracing the ending one has been 'given' makes such feelings precarious to express at best and at worst unacceptable to carers, family and hospice staff. The sense was that if one was unable to achieve a quick death then one must approach one's prolonged death in ways that alleviate the social sufferings of others; a departing gift of sorts. Yet, such 'gifts' are necessarily morally laden and, furthermore, they potentially make certain feelings and emotions almost incommunicable. As shown above and in the other interviews, these underlying feelings were expressed as stories of 'the good death' (see also Payne, Langley-Evans and Hillier 1996). While at times couched with statements like 'it's a bit selfish' and 'I know it would be traumatic for the family', these hypothetical deaths would remove the omnipresent burden of 'dying well' and the need to be virtuous in death.

## *'Being a Solid Brick': The Burden of Terminal Masculinities*

Feeling like a burden is regularly an important theme at the end of life, and furthermore, for some people it may form a key part of their reason for entering the hospice (McPherson, Wilson and Murray 2007; Murray et al. 2003). Similarly, in the interviews, feeling like a burden and the difficulties of accepting help were emphasised by the male participants. Lack of independence was a key theme, and so too was the incompatibility of 'the slow death' and the male identity:

> *Interviewer*: Um, how, what's it like accepting care, and help from people?

> *Participant* (male): Oh it's not easy, I'm not good at that, I'm not, I'm um, well I'm really hopeless at asking for help, just absolutely hopeless. And even then if people offer it, I contemplate what it is that they are offering, and what's my reverse commitment to this, is it actually helpful, does altruism really exist? … But yeah, I do have some difficulty accepting, asking for and accepting help.

Another respondent comments:

> *Participant* (male): Put it this way, nobody would ever say that they've, it's been their aim in life to get sick at the end of it and die in a certain particular way. I don't know, I can only put it from a male point of view, possibly, 'cause I know we men, and probably women too, to a great degree as well, we each of us all, we're all very proud of our own independence, our own abilities to, see ourselves through life, with ah, the provision of a roof over our head, and ah, bringing our children up, well fed and protected and sheltered, sort of thing. Owning your own home, it's sort of being a solid brick in the community sort of thing. So it's very, very hard when it comes to, when we start to get frail …

Another respondent comments:

> *Participant* (male): It's a macho thing … It's very hard to give up your independence. I should have got psychological help earlier but I couldn't ask for it.

The gendered character of dying and receiving care was clear in the interviews and the specific challenges end-of-life care presents within a wider context of the 'male role'. Related, in turn, to the typification of the heart attack as how men *should die*, gendered themes ran throughout the interviews with the men, uncovering the sense of masculine identity as being eroded by end-of-life and hospice care. While feeling like a burden and losing one's independence will impact across the spectrum of hospice patients, these results suggest that the impacts on some men may be even more acute. 'Being a solid brick in the community', rather than a person in need of help, encapsulated the desire of the men interviewed and the underlying grief of the loss of this status. One participant stated during the interview that he would like to take his own life if allowed. Another talked about the need for self-determination, even within the hospice, and the ethics of self-termination:

> *Participant* (male): I think they should have the same system as what the Dutch have, self-euthanasia, I believe in that, I think it should be like, you press a button and you say goodbye.
>
> *Interviewer*: The right to die.

> *Participant*: The right to die. I mean it's no good having people, it's no good shooting seven thousand dogs a year, which is what they do in [specific Australian State], and leaving the humans to suffer, you know, that to me is not right, that's what I think anyway.

While the desire to hasten death is by no means restricted to men (Kelly et al. 2002), and is not presented here as a mere artefact of masculine identity, there were subtle and important connections between talk around dying and the male identity. Specifically, a sense of social value and masculine potency was often topicalised by the men during the interviews, with the idealised death viewed as swift and even self-determined (see Kelly et al. 2002). Thus, while 'fighting on' was considered virtuous, 'ending it now' reflected a masculine form of potency and self-determination; a fitting end for a male not wishing to experience further erosion of the masculine self. Yet, not all the men felt this way about dying and there were alternative reflections of dying and being in the hospice:

> *Participant* (male): I'm in here [the hospice] now. But to be quite honest, I hope that, you know, that it is more an extended period than a short period. I suppose everyone hopes that. It's quite a normal reaction. That you want to, ah, last as long as you can. It's probably, it is absolute greed on the person's behalf … because you are wanting to extract that little bit more out of life, than what may be available, but anyway, we do our best, and that's basically it …

While the above respondent was, if you like, a 'negative case', his account reflects the importance of not imposing a linear model of the interplay between masculine identity and desire to hasten or self-determine death. Rather, gender identity is one element within the complex array of issues including identity, culture and interpersonal relationships.

## *Recognition and the Politics of Caring*

As noted above, there is an emerging literature on cancer and caring and forms of gendered emotional labour (Emslie et al. 2009; Thomas, Morris and Harman 2002), but no research within the hospice environment and from the position of those being cared for. Following Chattoo and Ahmad (2008), within the hospice context I do not present caring and dying as distinct dichotomous entities. Rather, and as talked about during the interviews, the carer–cared-for relationship is negotiated, embodied and temporal in character. Moreover, it is situated within a moral framework of ethical practice (that is, obligation, gift, reciprocity) and is often an unrecognised site of intense emotional labour. The interviewees expressed unanimous concern regarding the lack of social recognition for caring and the informal status of carers within the wider economies of end-of-life care:

> *Participant* (male): There is a lack of quality of life [at end of life], and the poor carer gets it as well … this is why I asked [my doctor] to put me in here … because I knew it would all fall on [wife's name] eventually, because they'll [health professionals] just let it all fall on top of her and hope that she can cope … [wife's name] is not even defined [by the State] as a carer, so she doesn't get anything.

Another respondent comments:

> *Participant* (male): Carers are the one's who are copping it at the moment, the Government's not supporting them very well. I mean ah, I think [wife] gets, caring for me, she gets about $90 a fortnight … it works out at about twenty-seven and a half cents an hour. [To get that] she's got to be able to prove that she has done twenty hours of actual physical hands-on … that she's got to prove. And nothing like, ah, going shopping, doing messages, that doesn't come into it … it's pretty hard to sort of make up that twenty hours …

Another respondent comments:

> *Participant* (male): They should support carers better [exclamation]. They try to get to a point, where they should know what's going on. When they got the old spaceship in the moon costing trillions of dollars. They couldn't spend a trillion dollars down here [hospice] in a bloody lifetime I bet. It's only politics, stinking rotten bloody politics …

The lack of recognition and support from the state for carers was a constant source of discontent in interviews. Health and social services were seen to implicitly rely on the emergence of a 'dedicated carer' to ensure adequate support is provided at the end of life. Yet, carers were often talked about as feeling unable to ask for help or financial support due to the more 'dire' situation of the person they were caring for. Furthermore, if they asked for help, financial structures and state policies were viewed as not capable of recognising the emotional labour of caring (James 1989), asking carers to justify the 'activities of caring' in order to receive financial and social support. In contrast to perceptions of government policy, caring was experienced as largely relational and emotional, rather than practical or instrumental (see Emslie et al. 2009 for the distinction between 'caring for' and 'caring about'). Problems caused by the bureaucratisation of dying and government attempts to quantify caring were particularly evident in their accounts, expressed as the lack of capacity to recognise the moral, inter-subjective and emotive character of caring and dying.

These accounts of the politics of caring and the state seem to reinforce classic sociological arguments about the problematic of the modern separation of values and economic transactions (Booth 1994). The moral economies of dying and caring seen here (gift, obligation and reciprocity) are more characteristic of much older community-oriented economies (Booth 1994; Sivaramakrishnan 2005). The problem occurs when these informal value systems and processes of reciprocity are not recognisable within a rational-legal bureaucratic system. Moral economists have long argued that this rupture has fundamentally disrupted ways of life that are structured around certain rights and ethics of reciprocity, loyalty and so on (Booth 1994).

## *Virtue, Mutual Obligation and the Gendering of Caring*

The caring–dying dynamic emerged as embedded in forms of moral practice and reciprocity within the interviews, with talk focusing on the centrality of mutual obligation in shaping the patient–carer relationship. While the interviewees often talked about their own willingness to 'rise to the challenge' at the end of life, they also talked about their carers as reciprocating through stoical and supportive dispositions. A clear gender theme also emerged within this relational framework of moral practice, this time in the accounts of the women interviewed who had male partners. They emphasised the centrality of gender scripts in shaping their carers' expressions of pain and suffering, and the practical and emotional traumas facing their carers as household gender dynamics broke down (see also Emslie et al. 2009). Stories of struggling to perform basic household tasks emerged, illustrating the embeddedness of caring within generationally-specific gender relations:

> *Participant* (female): He's always been very quiet and sort of laid back, he doesn't really say a lot, and it does bother me sometimes as to whether he's actually coping or not, and that was the reason I said that about going home, about making him not feeling as though he can't cope. Because that's the last thing I want for him. If he feels as though he can't cope, I would rather be in here, if that gives him a chance to come here spend some time, and then go home and get his head together ... And I do worry about him, because he's not really the sort of person to go out actively looking for help, he'll try and get through it himself.

Another respondent comments:

> *Participant* (female): Well at this stage I'm not really sure [how he is coping]. Um, because he's worried about the cooking side of it, which is really funny, because,

> you know, he's never cooked in his life. But I said, "Look, there's meals on wheels, I'm sure we can get that," I said, "There's frozen food" … he is worried … He's a man and he doesn't know how to do these things.

The interviews with the female participants provided insight into the male carer experience, including the gendering of the silent burden and lack of coping – a theme that flowed through each of the interviewees' accounts. Gender was viewed as critical in mediating carer experiences during the hospice stage, both in terms of willingness to ask for help and the kinds of struggles evident in the carers' everyday lives. Implicitly, caring emerged as incorporating elements of moral practice (responsibility and reciprocity) and emotional labour (management or suppression of emotions). Viewed by the participants as unwilling to reveal their suffering and pain, most felt their carers were performing 'stoicism' but were not coping underneath. Yet, there was recognition of the importance of their role (dying 'well') and the role of their carers (caring 'well') in coping with being and dying in the hospice.

It is important to note that the hospice itself was viewed as playing a critical role in ameliorating the obligations and pressures on carers. It was viewed as a key mechanism for alleviating silent suffering. The sense or recognition of 'carer burden' often formed at least part of the reason for deciding to enter the hospice rather than stay at home. The hospice staff were in turn viewed as highly successful in integrating and supporting carer needs, providing material and emotional support at key moments at the end of life:

> *Participant* (female): The fact that my husband could bring the dog in [to the hospice] is a big surprise! And the fact too that they, family can sleep over, that I hadn't expected. I mean I never thought of, I mean they bring out a fold-out bed. There is apparently another room over the other side that [family] can use. Of course, I couldn't have my husband in here, he'd keep me awake all night snoring! [laughs]

Another respondent comments:

> *Participant* (female): [They said], "Well, what are we going to do with you? What do you want to do? Do you want to go to a nursing home?", And I went, "No!". And they said, "Well," and I said, "Well what about the hospice?" And they said, "Well, yeah we can do that," and I said, "Well okay, we'll do that then." … And it was really good the way they got me in, cause they knew, what they knew was that [husband's name'] and I want to stay together, um, and that's why we wanted a room on our own, that we could put a bed in, and ah, that was the whole idea …

Another respondent comments:

> *Participant* (male): We came here so she wouldn't blow up at me. She needed a break, She's suffering too you know. She doesn't talk about it but she is.

A key advantage and strength of the hospice, as recounted by patients themselves, was its capacity to reduce the burden of dying and caring 'well'. It was talked about as giving relief and support at points when 'the good fight' was too hard. Furthermore, the hospice environment was perceived to embrace the carer in the process of dying (in very mundane but vital ways), providing an environment of community and inclusion. The hospice provided a means by which to alleviate the burden of being and doing 'the stoical carer' (allowing some space and emotional relief) while also allowing them to 'rise to the challenge'. As such, while their accounts reflected the challenges of mutual obligation even within the hospice, being in the hospice was seen to allow carers to 'get some time alone' and 'headspace', facilitating a feeling of much needed separateness once again. Ultimately, both caring and dying emerged as influenced, albeit differentially, by certain moral and gender scripts around death and dying, and the hospice interplayed with such dynamics, sometimes problematising and sometimes improving experiences at the end of life.

## Discussion

In this chapter I have highlighted some important elements of the contemporary hospice experience, identifying (at times gendered) understandings, expectations and interactional dynamics evident in this complex and emotive environment, particularly examining how *patients* themselves understand different forms of dying, and the assumptions underpinning their perspectives. As Clark (1990) previously observed, sociologists often use the language of reciprocity and exchange to analyse everyday interaction, but less commonly ask *why* people feel obligations within social relationships. Extending this argument further, I suggest that there is a need to explore, within different contexts, the limits to and factors shaping reciprocity and obligation. Certainly, the participants' articulated a relational ontology of dying as at least partially moral driven. What makes this a particularly moral dilemma is precisely that no 'good' choice is available, and yet one is expected to 'forge on' regardless (Frank 1997: 134). While the sense of obligation did emerge in their stories, it was more complex than a matter of subjugation to normative conceptions of 'dying well'. Patients' talk of dying and caring contained, produced and contested the notion of virtue (Chattoo and Ahmad 2008). Their stories revealed the importance of recognising and disentangling the intersectionality of moral practice and the self. Dying in a hospice, I argue, is shaped by the presence of normative understandings of 'the good death', but also complex personal and biographical factors. While 'rising to the challenge' was considered virtuous, it was in turn problematised within the context of some of the participants' gender identities. Being unable to maintain masculine status within the dying process emerged as important in the men's willingness to accept or perform 'the good fight'. The virtue of struggle was acknowledged, yet disintegrating masculine status and identity were incongruent with the broader sense of self. The perceived emotional and interpersonal cost of being a burden (of needing help) and the impotency of a drawn out death (being weak, sequestered and out of control) were central to the men's experiences of being in the hospice and dying.

Moral accountability is not transcendent, but rather develops through socio-cultural identities and divisions of labour that establish how responsibilities are shared and enacted (Mohammed and Peter 2009). What is necessary in the context of end-of-life care is a better understanding of how individuals negotiate moral framings and their situational applicability (Gordon 1990: 164). I am aware that some may perceive my focus on moral aspects of death and dying as regressive (see also Frank 1997). Yet, as indicated above and in previous chapters, my emphasis on caring and dying as forms of moral practice does not disallow human agency and self-determination. As Chattoo and Ahmad (2008) rightly posit, to conceptualise caring (or dying) as an 'infringement of autonomy', undermines their meaning and centrality in the negotiation of moral economy of self and identity. The moral practices of 'dying well' and 'caring well', and how these are done by different actors, reflect constraint *and* agency, choice *and* the pressures of normative values. The key, from my perspective, is to document how individual understandings, decisions and thought processes are influenced (often differentially) by different personal, interpersonal and cultural values and dynamics.

The importance of investigating caring from a different stakeholder perspective (not just those of carers themselves) was also evident in the interviews. While not often revealed in studies of carer accounts, the interviews reflected the potential for carers to accept the 'virtue' of suffering. Moreover, a perceived lack of recognition of carer suffering was emphasised, with accounts of ineffective state support systems incapable of recognising 'emotional labour' as a valid part of caring. This emotional work of caring and dying, on the part of carer and patient, was viewed as critical to being able to interact and live meaningfully within the hospice, but it was also hard work and needed relief, recognition and effective support systems. It was, as Exley and Letherby (2001) suggest, work for the other *and* on the self; it was neither altruistic nor unconditional, but rather situational, temporal and critical for the management of interaction, living and the self at the end of life.

Gender dynamics permeated the interviewees' accounts, featuring strongly in the interviews with both the male and the female participants in terms of caring and dying in the hospice. In particular, the gendered character of the caring–dying relationship was evident in the female participants' partners who were 'stoical' and yet struggled to 'do normal things'. This was situated within a socio-generational context of a household gendered division of labour and a breakdown in such dynamics at the end of life (see Emslie et al. 2009). The male carers were viewed as 'not coping' yet silent, due to a need to present an image of being 'able to cope'. Again, notions of manliness and not being seen to 'complain' pervaded the participants' accounts, illustrating the mediation of dying within a gendered form of relationality. Their accounts reflect, as Chattoo and Ahmad (2008) also observe, 'coping' as physical endurance and moral resilience. The virtues of caring and the persistence of silent suffering were evident. Yet, stoicism, while linked to cultural ideas about men and strength, was in turn evident in the men's representations of their wives[1] and partners. Thus, while gendered in nature, there were consistent themes around caring as moral practice across each of the interviews, particularly in relation to the need for an acknowledgement of carer pain and suffering.

In this chapter I provide insight into just some of the gendered and moral influences on experiences near death, and particularly within a hospice environment. What was particularly revealing was the interplay of ideas about dying (dying 'well') and ideas about the self (being a man) and how people negotiate these potentially competing cultural scripts and personal meanings in a very complex and emotive life stage. These accounts merely scratch the surface of what is a highly differentiated and rich area for research. As I also outline in more depth in the conclusion, biographically-driven research is needed to explore how other components of the self, including ethnicity, age and class, shape perceptions of 'good deaths', 'bad deaths' and all those in between. This would add another layer of sophistication to our understanding of the psycho-social and cultural processes operating within end-of-life care environments, and the potential impact these have on decision making and patient experiences near death. I now move to questions of the body, which interplay with gendered accounts of dying, including the embodied experience of being in end-of-life care.

---

1 All except one identified as being heterosexual and most had a partner or were married. While I do not wish to impose a normative conception of partnership and sexuality on these findings, drawing from the data, most identified within a traditional framework of heterosexual marriage or partnership.

# Chapter 9
# The Dying Body

## Introduction

The body has too often been sidelined in the sociology of health and illness. A focus on social structures and aggressively pursuing the *social* has contributed to a de-emphasis on *bodies* (Howson and Inglis 2001), including embodied experiences of illness and the dying process (Lawton 1998, 2002). According to Howson and Inglis (2001), sociologists have had to retrieve 'the body' because the development of the discipline has been premised on the Cartesian legacy: the ontological distinction between mind and body. The argument is that sociology had privileged the mind and rationality over the body (Howson and Inglis 2001: 298; see also Turner 1984). While other disciplines such as feminist studies and anthropology interrogated matters of the body, with some notable exceptions (for example, Hughes and Paterson 1997; Kelly and Field 1996; Shilling 2007, 2012; Scott and Morgan 1993; Turner 1984; Witz 2000), the sociology of health and illness only relatively recently began to directly address the nexus of corporeality and the social. Oddly enough, the tendency to not emphasise the body continues for social and behavioural research in palliative care and the end of life. With a few exceptions (for example, Glaser and Strauss 1966; Lawton 1998, 2002; Lofland 1976), there is a distinct lack of social research exploring embodied experiences of dying.

The palliative and hospice literature has tended to assume that the body is central at the end of life without actually exploring the social and cultural meanings ascribed to bodily decay, disintegration and loss of bodily control (see Lawton 1998, 2002 for an exception), but more specifically, without exploring social and cultural meanings of the embodied *and* bodily experience of dying, the implications for self and identity, and the relationship of embodied experiences to wider socio-cultural discontents. Dying is, at a very basic level, the ultimate (em)body(ied) experience: when the body stops functioning. To those working and caring in end-of-life settings the experience of dying is necessarily tied to bodies. Dying clearly articulates the interplay of the physiological, existential and social. It is *bodies out of order* while paradoxically playing out the *natural order* of things. It is also a curious contest between what *bodies do* (cellular death and bodily disintegration) and what *persons want* (often, although not always, life and longevity). Dying is thus the ultimate battle between the respective limits of, and co-dependencies between, physiology *and* personhood (Hockey, Komaromy and Woodthorpe 2010; Tullis 2012).

An emphasis on the body requires recognition of a range of cultural practices and shifts during the nineteenth, twentieth and now twenty-first centuries. Dying challenges an important project of modernity: the pursuit of human mastery over disease and thus control over the body (Shilling and Mellor 1996; Turner 1987), as outlined in the Introduction. Dying captures, or perhaps more accurately unsettles, a range of modern sensibilities toward sidelining, bettering or working the body (Davis 2013). Modern techniques of the body seek to delay the onset of ageing, decay and physical disintegration, and dying is the ultimate showdown between cultural expectations and physiological inevitability. Even when dying, we (and our formal and informal carers) embark on *body projects*. We are exposed to culturally important practices of disciplining our troubled and ill-disciplined bodies. This takes many forms including in the context of self-healing (see Chapter 7) as well as through hospital and hospices which offer increasingly potent (but ultimately failing) techniques and technologies for bodily and symptom control near death (see also Chapters 3 and 4).

I argue in this chapter that dying reveals much about our social and cultural understandings of and relationship to the body. Dying is inscribed with modern sensibilities toward bodily containment, mastery, cleanliness, sanitisation and so forth. These cultural dispositions can make dying an even more troubling experience for many people dying, and also to those accompanying people toward death. Dying fundamentally disorders particular embodied social relations and ritualised cultural performances of healthy bodies, often engendering repulsion and revulsion (at the self and at other selves). It involves a struggle to contain the body at the end of life. Through the accounts of people dying in the hospice environment, I explore such relations of fear, practices of resistance and relations of care as enmeshed in questions of the body.

## Background

### *The Sociology of the Body*

Scholars have made significant contributions to developing a renewed sociology of the body, including Turner (1984, 1987), Frank (1991), Shilling (2007, 2012), Williams and Bendelow (1998) among others. Their work has provided the opportunity to rethink a significant limitation of a rather disembodied field of the sociology of health and illness. This tendency at times reinforced the dualistic tendencies of the medical normativities being examined. Sociology, in over-privileging the social, disconnected its reflections on humanity from the body and embodied experiences (Morgan 1993; Burkitt 1999; see Nettleton 2010; Scott and Morgan 1993). As Howson and Inglis (2001: 298) argue, this meant an over-rationalisation of social life and a lack of emphasis on matters of the body. The resurgence in discussion of the body raised the threat that work focusing intently on bodies would facilitate a new form of reductionism which would be equally as problematic. Given this context, and following Howson and Inglis (2001: 298), I focus attention not on the body as *the* object of scrutiny, but rather orientate toward body matters in the dying process to add another layer of complexity to my analysis. This includes considering the body and embodied experiences as located within a particular social context (following Howson and Inglis 2001: 298). A discrete focus on the body lends itself toward reifying a dualistic framework. To disrupt this tendency, Howson and Inglis (2001: 303–4) reflect on the approach of Merleau-Ponty, offering a useful way of thinking about body *and* self (see also Crossley 1995) positing that the solution to this dualistic tendency is to show that human beings were neither purely 'minds' or 'subjects', referring to them as body-subjects (see Merleau-Ponty 1996). They argue for a 'fundamental existential condition whereby subjectivity and corporeality are wholly intertwined and indissociable, elements of the same elementary substance' (Howson and Inglis 2001: 303–4). In these terms, the body is subject and the subject is the body, with the distinction between body and subjectivity being an abstract theoretical notion (Kelly and Field 1996; Nettleton 2010; Shilling 2012). I intend to pursue such an approach in my analysis.

## *Bodies, Dying and the Abject*

The body as diseased and symptom producing has been well researched, with biomedical literature focusing on the medical solutions to physiological suffering at the end of life (for example, Sykes and Thorns 2003), and psychosocial research focusing on the cognitive-behavioural and psychotherapeutic possibilities for easing people through the end of life (for example, Price and Hotopf 2009). Mostly the focus has not been on the perception, reception and cultural meanings of bodies or the embodied experience of dying, with some notable exceptions (for example, Lawton 1998; Waskul and van der Riet 2002; Whitaker 2010). Lawton (2001), as mentioned previously, provided a novel and challenging examination of how people experience dying in an institutional setting – and as an embodied experience – arguing that institutions sequester the dying body or person (see also Froggatt 2001; Hockey, Komaromy and Woodthorpe 2010; Morris and Thomas 2005). Interesting questions for me in this context are: What underlies the cultural desire to sequester dying people and their troubling bodies? What do their bodies do? How do they make us and them feel? How may that prompt a desire within us to sideline or sequester them and their bodies? And what practices do we utilise to achieve this?

The basis of the practice of sequestering, as seen in accounts of those who are dying, lies in the unique challenges dying bodies pose culturally to many of us. The problematic of the cultural reception of dying bodies (and their symptomatology) informs both self-perception of one's dying body, as well as how dying bodies are received by others. Who cares for the dying and where they care for them also heavily inflects the embodied dying process. Where dying bodies are located, whether in a hospice or at home, fundamentally shapes the possibilities and problems of the body. Moreover, what is social and culturally acceptable for *bodies to do* heavily influences where and how we die. Entrance into the hospice, for example, may be a result of individuals or families not being able to cope with various bodily problems (such as symptoms, pain or incontinence). Thus, the cultural reception of dying bodies is central to the contemporary experience of dying and caring for the dying.

One relevant conceptual line of argument in making sense of dying bodies is that of Kristeva (1982), who in *The Powers of Horror* outlines cultural sensibilities in and around waste and filth – the politics and moralities of abjection. Utilising this frame of reference, dying is about the cultural reception of increasingly compromised and disordered bodies, and much of the reception of dying lies within cultural dynamics around decay, hygiene, cleanliness, control and disgust. These culturally-specific scripts are critical to understanding the embodied experience of dying (and caring for the dying). Regarding the culturally improper or unclean, Kristeva states:

> Loathing an item of food, a piece of filth, waste, or dung. The spasms and vomiting that protect me. The repugnance, the retching that thrusts me to the side and turns me away from defilement, sewage, and muck. The shame of compromise, of being in the middle of treachery. The fascinated start that leads me toward and separates me from them. (Kristeva 1982: 2)

*Continues*:

> … without makeup or masks, refuse and corpses *show me* what I permanently thrust aside in order to live. These body fluids, this defilement, this shit are what life withstands, hardly and with difficulty, on the part of death. There, I am at the border of my condition as a living being. My body extricates itself, as being alive, from that border. Such wastes drop so that I might live, until, from loss to loss, nothing remains in me and my entire body falls beyond the limit – *cadere*, cadaver. If dung signifies the other side of the border, the place where I am not and which permits me to be, the corpse, the most sickening of wastes, is a border that has encroached upon everything. (Kristeva 1982: 3)

These excerpts on the nature of abjection have much relevance to the experiences of dying bodies (and caring for dying people and their bodies). Much of the *act* of dying involves the increasing prominence of an unbridled and out-of-control body that can no longer contain its edges. The body is no longer able to hold its fluids and perform tight boundaries between the sanitised exterior and the repugnant interior (Kristeva 1982). This is clearly illustrated below in the interview data I present. The body's waste, supposed to be washed away in ritualised private moments (defecation), moves in unsettling ways into other spheres of social interaction, requiring 'expert' or 'professional' input to contain the body's increasingly immoral boundaries (cf. Waskul and van der Riet 2002). In this way dying represents the fundamental disruption of well-established borders. A coherent bordered body reinforces the security of self and personhood, as contained within stable moral physical boundaries, and a clear border lies between the self, life, our environment, others and what is clean/dirty, alive/dead, contained/uncontained. Disruption of this border compromises the security of personhood. Kristeva notes, in relation to abjection:

> It is no longer I who expel, "I" is expelled.
>
> The border has become an object. How can I be without border? That elsewhere that I imagine beyond the present, or that I hallucinate so that I might, in a present time, speak to you, conceive of you – it is now here, jetted, abjected, into "my" world. Deprived of world, therefore, *I fall in a faint.* In that compelling, raw, insolent thing in the morgue's full sunlight, in that thing that no longer matches and therefore no longer signifies anything, I behold the breaking down of a world that has erased its borders: fainting away. The corpse, seen without God and outside of science, is the utmost of abjection. It is death infecting life. Abject. It is something rejected from which one does not part, from which one does not protect oneself as from an object. Imaginary uncanniness and real threat, it beckons to us and ends up engulfing us. (Kristeva 1982: 4)

Waskul and van der Riet (2002) provide an important explication of the issue of the abject in the context of dying of cancer. They argue that the out-of-control abject body threatens the order between bodies and selves, contesting the normal 'mastery of the body'. The abject body, they argue, threatens the order between bodies and others. They add to this various typologies of the abject including leaky, grotesque and repulsive bodies, arguing for a threatened order in dying, making public our normally private purging of what lies inside (faeces, blood, urine). This work provides an important way into understanding dying as bound to matters of the body, and its cultural reception/production. In dying, and as embodied actors, we break down many of the ritual boundaries of social life, producing, as Waskul and van der Riet (2002) posit, humiliating moral connotations. This provides a rich series of insights to which I would add the practice of bodily resistance. Drawing on aspects of the notion of the body-subject and the notion of abjection, I consider how we treat and experience disordered bodies at the end of life, practices of resistance to the final acts of the body, social relations of fear and horror, and the dynamics of receiving care in the context of bodily disintegration.

## Into the Field

### *Bodies Out of Order*

I return once again to my research in an in-patient hospice in New South Wales, Australia, and focus on participant accounts of their 'failing' and 'dying' bodies. These accounts illustrate the experience of their collapsing bodies and how the swift decline of bodily boundaries can be experienced in palliative and hospice care settings. These accounts are situated within a struggle for continued bodily integrity and abhorrence for bodily disintegration. Some participants began their reflections from an earlier point in life and others began with the experience of dying in the hospice:

> *Participant*: … people are going well until their, early to middle fifties, you know, coping with things, even though they realise they're getting older and they can't do things they used to do twenty years ago, but then all of a sudden there's a period, and in a couple of years just, everything falls off, together, you know?… and all of a sudden, you know, things are bogging down, the kidneys are playing up, your liver's giving you trouble … and ah, your teeth are falling out, you've got a peptic ulcer there somewhere, you know, "Aw, look at me legs, the bloody varicose veins, Aaww"! You know, and all of this kind of thing, and it can happen very quickly. [male]

Another respondent:

> *Participant*: No, no, I was, I was dead in the water [before coming into the hospice]. My equipment's bloody, can't do things. Mainly I couldn't walk and I was weak, and I've always been a fairly strong person, you know, able to do things. [Male]

Another respondent:

> *Participant*: This [paralysis from advanced cancer] has only happened in the last month … [I was] virtually paralysed by half past seven on the Saturday morning. I could feel tingling in my right foot, and by about two or three o'clock by the

> afternoon, I was paralysed right up to the waist … 'cause of all the medication I was on they were trying to control the pain. I was constipated. I was only in there, well I went in there on the early Tuesday morning and on the Saturday morning this happened, by three o'clock I couldn't walk. I was operated on at eight o'clock on the Sunday morning and I was brought over here [to the hospice] last Monday … That photo on the wall there [standing up and healthy], was taken … less than three months ago. [Male]

Captured acutely in the participant's photo he showed me of his body three months prior to being in the hospice (walking and 'healthy'), the diagnosis of metastatic prostate cancer and subsequent spinal metastases meant that his physiological capacity was dramatically reduced. He went from 'well' to 'terminal' in a matter of weeks. His body – spine and bowel in particular – was disintegrating causing huge distress. The dramatic contrast between his recent embodied self and his current debilitated body was experienced as humiliating, impotent and depression inducing. The horror 'of someone having to wipe my arse' and having 'no control over my bowel' was palpable in the interview, with a desperation evident around having lost bodily potency and control. He was 'repulsed' at the faecal matter that surrounded him through no bowel control, despondent at his seemingly healthy body's steep decline to total disintegration.

The medicalisation and institutionalisation of dying attempts to facilitate some level of bodily control with technologies and medications used within the hospice to instil some sense of order on these participants' bodies, and to impose 'natural' and 'normal' rhythms on their dying bodies. While one 'variable' may be controlled (sleep or pain) others were talked about as impossible to control (urination or defecation). With only a partial reconstitution of order there was a constant tension between projects for maintaining bodily 'normalcy' and recognising their bodies were in fact 'out of order' and unable to be disciplined. A participant and their carer talked about their (and the hospice's) attempts to instil a 'normal' sleep pattern:

> *Carer*: … since she's been having these sleeping pills …
>
> *Interviewer*: It's made a difference [to her sleep in the hospice]?
>
> *Carer*: Well, she bombs out ...
>
> *Interviewer*: Yeah?
>
> *Carer*: … she goes to sleep … I mean a couple of times she's woken me up at four o'clock in the morning, still under the influence of these tablets, you know, she can't string a sentence together …

> *Interviewer*: Yeah?
>
> *Carer*: … and um, I said to her one morning, "Do you need changing?" I felt around and she absolutely did need changing! She was saturated.
>
> *Participant*: I was saturated! But I didn't know it. [Female]

Above we see a husband and wife talking about the attempts to instil rest and sleep in the last few days of life. The participant died the following day. It illustrates the problematic of the out-of-control dying body. Despite medical attempts at imposing order, her body resisted, and order could not be maintained. While sleep is imposed the body continues to express its disorder – or the natural order of dying (in the last few weeks and days of life a 'normal' sleep pattern is unlikely to occur).

### *Horror in the Hospice: The Fear of Others and Others' Fear*

The hospice patients regularly talked about how their bodies and symptoms (for example, sounds, sights and smells of dying) impacted on visitors including family and friends. They talked of their and the hospice staff attempts to provide a reasonable 'frontstage' that was acceptable to visitors. While their partners were largely privy to the problems of their dying bodies, the body presented significant potential for trauma and horror for friends and family (including their own children). The hospice invested considerable time and energy, as reported in the interviews, in preparing them for visits from others, ensuring it was the optimal time of day, the optimal pain relief and that they were not 'struggling' in front of those who were visiting. The interviewed participants largely supported this, as they were acutely aware of the fear and horror their situation could conjure up and how this might result in fewer visits or upset people (and thereby upset them). With phrases like 'they can't see me like this', 'they can come back when I'm at my best' and so forth, the participants described a constant battle to present the most contained and controlled dying body possible, to sanitise the process of dying and keep the particularly difficult, unsettling and compromising events for private suffering and support from hospice staff.

> *Participant*: … Nothing could be worse then, like … when I run out of breath, and I probably don't look too good when I'm hacking and coughing, and trying to get my breath back, and getting rid of something up the airways and things like that, and it probably is not a pretty sight … one of our friends young daughters, she was about 12 or 13 at the time, she came to see me one day, it was the first time she'd seen me have a bit of trouble, and she got very upset

> about it … what you're seeing at the moment is only the tip of the iceberg, sort of thing, please don't be frightened about it, because that would upset me more than what I already am … sooner or later I won't be here, it's nothing to be afraid of …. [male]

The above interview excerpt provides insight into a concern across each of the participants' accounts: the potential of frightening and alienating family and friends, and in turn, their own moral responsibility to minimise distress and horror. Not 'scaring everyone' and 'making them feel worse than they already are' was an important aspect of the moral practice of hiding the disordered body. Consistent with some of Lawton's (1998) observations, the hospice reinforced such practices, encouraging a moral performance of acceptable dying, and removing or preventing interactions that might induce disgust or horror in others. In this sense, the embodied experience of dying was, once again, a moral project that was about containing and controlling the body as far as technology, expertise and individual stoicism could allow. Placing the responsibility for competent bodily performances on the individual, augmented by expert encouragement and input from formalised care facilities, is a particularly Western sensibility. Such fears and expectations of bodily mastery (self or relational) were viewed as both a benefit of hospice care (assistance in orchestrating body performances) and a limitation (struggle to not induce horror or forms of disgust). I return to this later in relation to hospice formal care and relations of disgust.

### *Body Projects: The 'Good Fight' and Resistance*

The modern sensibility of the body-as-project, and a constant resistance to 'natural' bodily processes including ageing, continues throughout the life course until death. While anti-ageing treatment bears no similarity to bodily practices within the hospice, they do share some important moral sensibilities. These include the desire to remain 'intact', 'contained', 'bordered' and 'stable'. There is a bodily-derived ethic evident in accounts of dying in a hospice which was often manifest in the interviews in relation to food or sleep. These body projects were as much about resisting dying as they were about retaining a recognisable bodily form. To retain a 'healthy looking' body was important and the shrinking or disappearing body was the source of much distress. It signified a lost battle of the mind over the body – the participants' own dualistic language – and was situated within a dynamic of resistance to what the body was doing (statements included 'I won't succumb', 'I'm not ready', 'I'm not going to let it [my body] get worse'). This resulted in an inevitable (losing) battle between the body and the self. The lack of an explanation for bodily transgressions (like incontinence, sleeplessness, coughing, weight loss) on the part of the hospice added significant frustrations. From a participant perspective they wanted explanations for *why* their bodies were acting up in these ways. From a hospice perspective, the body/person was in the process of dying, and so no specific explanation was necessary. In the interviews this resulted in persistent frustration with the unexplainable body in terms of its reactions and responses at this point in illness. Dying, as recounted by these participants, involved an embodied sense of slowly disappearing, but also a troubling disjunction between body and self. As Kristeva (1982) stated, the very experience of the dying body fundamentally contests the modern sense of 'I', the contained explainable body which does what it is meant to, which expresses healthy bordered relations with Others. Several participants talked about the lack of answers around what their bodies were doing, and frustrations with losing a healthy normal aesthetic:

> *Participant*: I feel that they [the hospice] haven't got enough answers. I feel that they haven't got enough answers, to, like I'm cough, cough, coughing and they don't seem to be able to understand why I'm cough, cough, coughing. They think it's because the cancer of the lungs, but um, surely there's something to stop me from doing the cough, cough, cough, cough, coughing? [Male]

Another respondent:

> *Participant*: I eat everything they give to me because I actually lost a lot of weight, I have to try and ... There's nothing of me, I looked at my body in the mirror last night and I said, "My God, where has it gone?" Yeah [my body] it's disappeared, so I'm eating now, plenty of food. [female]

Another respondent:

> *Participant*: I just have to be careful that I don't overdo it, and I have to keep eating. 'Cause I only weigh 40 kilos now. I eat quite a lot of food. [female]

Another respondent:

> *Participant*: … I'm not, I refuse to, I'm not ready to. I'm not ready to die yet. If it happens, it happens, you can't do anything about that … But while I can keep it at bay … the medication's been cut right down, which was really good, 'cause I went down from like thirty odd tablets a day, I'm down to about eight, 'cause they cut out a lot, a lot of the tablets I was taking. [female]

While a number of the participants had essentially released control of their body and symptomatology to the hospice, others were embarking on significant practices of resistance to what they saw as their unruly bodies. Considering *dying* was not often explicitly discussed in the hospice, it is unsurprising that there was a lot of talk of mysterious symptoms and bodily responses. Some participants aggressively did not want to die and were engaging in practices – whether increasing food or reducing medications – in order to instil some sense of control over their bodies. It is a dualistic notion but one that was strong in their accounts. There was anger at their weak bodies; they were in some respects separating themselves from the problems of their body, but also engaging in practices to regain control over them.

### *Bodies, Care, Dignity, Disgust*

The embodied experience of the hospice is relationally negotiated and inscribed, with both informal and formal carers shaping how matters of the body are dealt with. I have reflected on how visits from friends and family were managed to minimise the horror of exposure to unruly bodies. Embodied relations with formal carers (mainly hospice nursing staff) were in turn embedded in notions of bodily boundaries, control and personal responsibility for mastery. Even in the nursing context, moral scripts operated around responsibilities and norms of bodily performance. This included normative ideas about what was acceptable for a patient to do in the context of exercising bodily control (within the limits of their disease). The nurses were talked about as (at times) being repulsed by dying bodies and avoiding dealing with particular bodily or individual dysfunctions. Those who had little or no control over their defecation felt particularly marginalised and that their moral performances in dying were inadequate for the nursing staff. They were failing to exert control over a basic human function and ritual activity (of which timing and place of delivery is vital). The experience, often recounted by the partners in the interviews, was experienced as one of punishment for the disordered uncontrolled body, even if not intended by the staff:

> *Husband*: … one of the younger nurses went crook at her for making a mess in the bed, and I said, "Well nobody came to me when I pressed the buzzer!"… and you can only hang on so long.
>
> *Interviewer*: You can't go [to the toilet] on demand, can you?
>
> *Participant*: No … it just happens. [female]
>
> *Husband*: Especially if you're someone who's a bit incontinent and you're asleep, and you don't realise that you're doing it.

Another respondent:

> *Wife*: He [patient] buzzed [the nurses] because he noticed he was dirty in the bed, and what was it? An hour or more later before somebody came and changed him. How's his bedsores ever going to get better?
>
> *Participant*: That's like one day I buzzed them because I can't feel when I do a poo, but I can smell it [in the bed] … by the time that they got out here, I could see it out past my penis, you know … But it's not that they don't check it, they don't do anything about it.[male]

Another respondent:

> *Participant*: They've [nurses] got to learn [to deal with it] ... I mean, one came in here one afternoon, and the girl said, "Do you want to go to the toilet, darl?" And I said, "Yeah," … And the new girl's standing in the corner … and I said to her, "Why don't you get in there and help mate?", "No, I'm right here, this'll do me," … they just chuck you all around like a rag doll, they don't care about you … [I've] woken up at two o'clock, they put these, where you wipe [your bottom], and you can see these now, they've all gone down to buggery, that's the fluid in my bowel there … They don't touch [that area], unless I ask them, and then they just go flip, flop, flap and that's it. [male]

While it is important to bear in mind the potential for atrocity stories in these participants' accounts – that sometimes things do go wrong in the hospice and that this may not be reflective of a lot of care received in these settings – these accounts raise some interesting dynamics around care, responsibility and expectations of bodily control. The construction of 'good' and 'bad' or 'credible' patients has been well documented within the palliative care literature, as mentioned previously, but not so in relation to bodily responses, and associated bodily performances. Further research on how sensibilities around disgust, abjection and repulsion creep into formalised care relationships is warranted, including how failure in bodily control and specific symptomatologies may contribute to the construction of disorderly patients. It would seem likely that the nurses were in fact expressing wider cultural discontents around bodily control and mastery, and that such ideas were operating within the context of end-of-life care.

## Discussion

Questions around dying and a distinctly embodied experience are many and I have touched on only a few key issues. The issues I have chosen here are: relations of disorder; the fear of horror; resistance in the form of body projects; and how body matters inflect care. Each of these emerge from the troubling character of the dying body – its decay, its smells, its excretions and its lack of conformity to what we understand and want the body or person to act like. The dying body presents the individual with considerable moral dilemmas and normative frameworks in order to contain their body. The dying body loses form, its excretions compromise ritual practices, and in doing so it conjures up fear (in the person and in the audience). The hospice, on one level, provides a means of managing this disordered situation, but also lacks the capacity to provide for disorder. When 'natural' sleep is imposed at night, there is 'unnatural' sleep in the day. The hospice facilitates a limited but still potent way of containing the quickly disintegrating body.

The hospice staff themselves were not always experienced by the participants as immune from the cultural sensibilities of, and desires for, bodily integrity – labour cannot be disconnected from cultural practices. From these accounts, in the course of caring the hospice staff perpetuate a sense of responsibility for bodily control and (limited) mastery. This was governed through the construction of 'good' and 'bad' patients, and approaches to care within the hospice (see also Chapters 3 and 4). Whether dying person, family or formal carer, it was clear that the dying body troubled relations even in the hospice, polluting and contaminating established norms and boundaries. Dying offended sensibilities – of the person and of those surrounding them – resulting in a battle against the disorderly body, furthering a dualistic split between self and body. The body was giving up, but the milieu encouraged 'battle' and the presentation of a (partially) ordered self. In this sense, the embodied experience is one containing disorder, disgust, resistance and the normativity of an ethic of control. Moreover, the protection of the dirty secret, that the taken-for-granted boundaries of life/bodies were being broken down, and ritual practices compromised, was enabled by the hospice in many respects.

In some respects these interviews brought up more questions than answers in terms of the body. I often considered whether what I was observing and hearing were merely 'natural' struggles, 'normal' tensions and that dying inevitably involved frustrations, resistance and repulsion regarding the body. That in fact, at any point in recent history, had I interviewed people who are dying (taking into account the variations presented by individual biographies) they would have raised similar issues. Yet, there were subtle influences at play here that make their experiences revealing of the evolving character of dying and 'treatment' of the body – the collective ways in which we view and manage dying bodies. They revealed both persistent struggles with the dying body and new intersections of bodies, institutions and expertise. Moreover, that in end-of-life contexts, attempts to *ease* the body to death is a culturally meaningful, and in turn potentially problematic, process. While many people enter hospices due to the need for assistance around symptomatology and 'bodily issues' (bearing in mind all the social influences on tolerability outlined in previous chapters), and the institution offers some amelioration, the body's/person's unruly behaviour continues. For me, the outcome of my observations around this topic within the hospice was that *perceptions* of the body – as 'weak', 'disappearing', 'repulsive', 'lacking control', 'unnatural', 'borderless' and 'revolting' to others – cause significant additional suffering. How this plays out across cultures, gender identities and according to social class is an area for future inquiry.

# Chapter 10
# Conclusion

## The Importance of Understanding Dying as a Social Occasion

Numerous scholars prior to this book have laid the foundations for understanding dying as a distinctly social occasion, rather than merely as a biophysical event (e.g. Clark 1993; Glaser and Strauss 1968; Hockey 1990; Howarth 2007b; Kellehear 1990, 2007, 2009; Seale 1998a). In this sense, I am not introducing anything particularly new by emphasising some of the social and cultural dynamics surrounding the end of life. However, as social and cultural changes occur, the dynamics of dying, as well as the structural, social, political, professional and economic influences on care and illness also change. Some of these changes which I have explored within this book include shifts in: professional dynamics and identities (for example, between medicine and nursing); rising public awareness of the dying process and care practices therein (for example, greater exposure to palliative care); and the institutional processes and forms of care offered (for example, expansion of specialist palliative care services). Moreover, in recent decades there has been a distinct series of social shifts, including sites of weakening kinship ties, processes of secularisation, the rise of neoliberalism, enhanced migration and population diversity, contraction of the welfare state and increased privatisation of healthcare. These sites of social change in turn shape the experience of illness and dying, necessitating ongoing analysis in order to understand and, in some cases, respond to the changing landscapes of the end of life.

Underpinning my analysis throughout this book has been the development of a better understanding of the potential *constraints* placed upon various actors in the context of contemporary dying, particularly in institutional settings – what I would call the evolving, culturally-located normativity of dying. In developing this analysis I have sought to unpack how a range of normative influences manifest in human actions and are evident in the lived experience of dying and how social beliefs and structures limit and enable certain actions at the end of life. My analysis of doctors and nurses centred on how their work is situated (often implicitly) within forms of emotion, subtle cultural logics and evolving but persistent professional power structures, and on how health professionals struggle to balance the requirements of professional objectivity alongside the relational pressures and social influences in their everyday work. In this way I have sought to reveal end-of-life 'labour' as situated within, but often unreflective of, social pressures and moral frameworks. What makes *the social* important is that it is concurrently driving clinical decisions and therapeutic trajectories, yet it is often concealed in everyday clinical work. By revealing the relational components of establishing medical futility and acknowledging dying, I hope to work toward a view of *emotional reflexivity* as a core part of medical and nursing work, rather than something that is sidelined by the conveying of technical information and medical or nursing knowledge.

In examining individual experiences of dying and carers' accounts therein, the critical message I have tried to weave through the previous chapters is that there are *persistent tensions* around *choice* and relations of *obligation* at the end of life. As becomes clear from my examination of the hospice, what a critical sociological investigation reveals is that relations of informal care *and* formalised care contain, perpetuate and reify certain ways of dying, *asking* for certain things and even *demanding of people* particular types of endings. Of course, such institutional structures and social relations are concurrently enabling and constraining, thus offering a contradictory series of social and care relations which are in turn situated within individual circumstances. What is entirely consistent across the patient accounts I have had the privilege to hear over the last decade is that dying is a precarious culmination of divergent interests – and that such interests are not necessarily revealed, addressed or given recognition pre or peri the end of life. While this could be said about most social situations, the distinct problem lies in the fact that certain ways of being (such as rejecting 'terminality' and pursuing survival, or, refusing to 'accept' death) are ascribed certain levels of interpersonal legitimacy, and through relations of illegitimacy, potentially disallow or reduce personal dignity. Individuals can be thus framed within particular moralities of dying (cf. Fraser 1995), with indignity manifest in a sense of moral failure on the part of those who are dying to meet the standards and norms regarding what is good, right appropriate and desirable (cf. Wong and Tsai 2007). Alternatively, there exists unnecessary fixation on survival with subsequent suffering resulting from the moral frameworks surrounding the dying person (vis-à-vis individual preference). Some may well say, there will always be moralities operating within any given social context, and moral frameworks are not a priori problematic. Indeed, I do not propose a relativist stance. What I propose is greater transparency in relations of power, influence and obligation within the spaces where increasingly people are dying in contemporary societies, and for greater reflectiveness around how powerful relational forces shape people's experiences near death. There are numerous issues and questions that I have not covered in this book and below I outline some key areas which I view as crucial next steps in the sociology of dying.

## Reflections on a Future Research Agenda for Sociological Research on Dying

### *A Focus on Dying Across Cultures*

One of the limitations of the analysis presented in this book is its focus on two OECD and Commonwealth countries whose health systems and level of socioeconomic development are largely consistent and indeed high by global standards. It remains the case that the most significant need in the development of palliative and end-of-life care services lies in the developing world, not OECD countries (Sepúlveda et al. 2002). Whilst I have outlined some of the problems manifest in these two western economically privileged contexts, including lack of community engagement or understanding of palliative care, significantly greater problems lie in the developing world. I have touched on a range of key issues in developing countries in recent work on cancer care in India (see Broom, Doron and Tovey 2009; Broom and Doron 2012; Broom and Doron 2013) where palliative and end-of-life care are non-existent in many geographical areas, and grossly misunderstood and stigmatised in many others. On the other hand, in India and in other developing nations there remain interesting potential angles of enquiry around the persistence of traditional beliefs systems around death and dying, and the potential intersections between medical expertise at the end of life and cultural values (see Doron and Broom 2011; and also Webster, Lacey and Quine 2007). Given the 'epidemiological transition' in the burden of disease occurring across the developing world, there is an urgent need to explore the social and cultural dynamics of dying in such transitional cultural contexts. Societies are highly differentiated in the extent to which economic development shapes the retention of beliefs and values and also in the use of traditional health practices, suggesting that approaches to dying will vary across time, space and culture.

### *The Biographical Mediation of Dying: Class, Ethnicity and Geography*

Another area of considerable priority for research into dying and end-of-life care is the dynamics of biographies in shaping experiences of dying. While I have only briefly touched on some of the biographical 'determinants' of dying – in relation to masculinities and gender identities – this is an important area of future inquiry. Just as Howarth (2007c) writes of the neglect of 'social class' in thinking about dying, so too have cultural diversity (Broom et al. 2013), geography (Castleden et al. 2010) and to a certain extend gender (Broom 2012b) been neglected in terms of thinking about the social dynamics and experiences of dying. Whether shaping proximity to care, or preparedness to engage in care, it is vital that we provide a contemporary understanding of the lived experience of more marginalised populations in our conceptions of dying as a social occasion. At the time of writing this book, in collaboration with colleagues I have embarked on new studies in this very area. This new program involves a mapping exercise with the premise that dying can be highly diversified across cultures and societies, and that care practices and service providers must be receptive to diverse needs and experiences (Oliviere, Monroe and Payne 2011).

### *Place, the Diminishing Welfare State, and Access to Informal Care*

While I have touched on socioeconomic constraints and issues around access to informal care, there is much to explore in this major area of social change. The rise in specialised palliative care in OECD countries has been recently accompanied by the tightening of public healthcare services and a move to the political right (with enhanced healthcare privatisation) in many nation states. Much like the case already in highly privatised systems (like the US), we will gradually see dying as increasingly reflective of structural conditions and opportunities emergent from forms of polarisation resulting from greater privatisation. While 'place of death' is often considered as related to personal preference – that is, where people wish to die – opportunities for particular deaths will be increasingly tied to private insurers and structural inequalities, which will thus mediate place of death and in turn experiences of dying.

Despite the majority of Australians not dying at home (around 14 per cent at the time of writing), informal care remains a crucial aspect of preparing for the end of life, although it is very much an artefact of opportunity and capacity. With reductions in state welfare and increases in cost of living (and longer working hours, with lower work security) the very character of informal care will be strained and challenged by already weakening kinship ties in the context of modernity. Inequities will be enhanced by differences in access to and experiences of informal care as pressures on family life continue to change kinship relations and ties. Wealthier families will have greater capacity for informal care, and greater capacity to cover for periods of time doing informal care and on bereavement leave.

### *Dying and Diversity*

While the focus in this book has been placed on cancer, the character of dying and its diversification must be a part of new research. Emerging issues, such as the specialised palliative care needs across illness contexts (e.g. HIV, heart failure, neurodegenerative diseases) as well as the associated social scripts surrounding different conditions, will be an important area of investigation. Mapping the end of life across different illnesses and dying contexts, and unpacking the social environments which people are exposed to, will be critically important aspects of future work in this area.

Each of the abovementioned themes place an emphasis on issues of social justice and potential disadvantage. Disadvantage and availability of opportunities in dying are probably the most pressing issues for sociologists currently working in this area. The key for future social research will be systematically documenting emerging structures of inequality and understanding the end of life as stratified and evolving rather than linear. This will require large-scale studies mapping the relationships between dying and biographies/demographics, as well as small-scale in-depth qualitative studies exploring the meaning and experience of dying in different contexts. This will facilitate a better understanding of the varied ways that people die and how we may improve this experience.

# References


Ablett, J.R. and Jones, R. (2007) Resilience and well-being in palliative care staff. *Psycho-Oncology* 16(8), 733–40.

Adamle, K. and Ludwick, R. (2005) Humor in hospice care: Who, where, and how much? *American Journal of Hospice and Palliative Care* 22(4), 287–90.

Ahmed, N., Bestall, J., Ahmedzai, S., Payne, S., Clark, D. and Noble, B. (2004) Systematic review of the problems and issues of accessing specialist palliative care by patients, carers and health and social care professionals. *Palliative Medicine* 18(6), 525–42.

Allen, D. (2001) Narrating nursing jurisdiction: 'Atrocity stories' and 'boundary-work'. *Symbolic Interaction* 24(1), 75–103.

Aoun, S. (2004) *The Hardest Thing We Have Ever Done: The Social Impact of Caring for Terminally Ill People in Australia.* Deakin West: Palliative Care Australia.

Aoun, S., Kristjanson, L., Hudson, P., Currow, D. and Rosenberg, J. (2005) The experience of supporting a dying relative: Reflections of caregivers. *Progress in Palliative Care* 13(6), 319–25.

Ardelt, M. and Koenig, C.S. (2006) The role of religion for hospice patients and relatively healthy older adults. *Research on Ageing* 28(2), 184–215. DOI: 10.1177/0164027505284165.

Armstrong, N. (2007) Discourse and the individual in cervical cancer screening. *Health* 11(1), 69–85.

Arnold, R.L. and Egan, K. (2004) Breaking the 'bad news' to patients and families. *American Journal of Geriatric Cardiology* 13(6), 307–12.

Back, A.L., Young, J.P., McCown, E., Engelberg, R.A., Vig, E.K., Reinke, L.F. and Curtis, J.R. (2009) Abandonment at the end of life from patient, caregiver, nurse, and physician perspectives. *Archives of Internal Medicine* 169(5), 474–79.

Bailey, C., Murphy, R. and Porock, D. (2011) Professional tears: Developing emotional intelligence around death and dying in emergency work. *Journal of Clinical Nursing* 20(23–24), 3364–72.

Baklinski, T. (2009). *Pope Benedict XVI: Euthanasia is a false solution to the drama of suffering.* http://www.euthanasia.com/benedictsolution.html.

Baltes, P.B. and Smith, J. (2003) New frontiers in the future of ageing: From successful ageing of the young old to the dilemmas of the fourth age. *Gerontology* 49(2), 123–35.

Barrett, B., Marchand, L., Scheder, J., Plane, M.B., Maberry, R., Appelbaum, D., Rakel, D., and Rabago, D. (2003) Themes of holism, empowerment, access, and legitimacy define complementary, alternative, and integrative medicine in relation to conventional biomedicine. *Journal of Alternative and Complementary Medicine* 9(6): 937–47.

Beck, U. and Beck-Gernsheim, E. (1996) Individualization and 'precarious freedoms'. In Heelas, P., Lash, S. and Morris, P. (eds), *Detraditionalization*. Oxford: Blackwell, pp. 23–48.

Beck, U. and Beck-Gernsheim, E. (2001) *Individualization: Institutionalized Individualism and its Social and Political Consequences*. London: Sage.

Becker, E. (1973) *The Denial of Death*. New York: Free Press.

Beilin, R. (1981) Social functions of denial of death. *OMEGA Journal of Death and Dying* 12(1), 25–35.

Bell, K. (2009). 'If it almost kills you that means it's working': Cultural models of chemotherapy expressed in a cancer support group. *Social Science & Medicine* 68(1), 169–76.

Bell, K. (2010). Cancer survivorship, mor(t)ality, and lifestyle discourses on cancer prevention. *Sociology of Health and Illness* 32(3), 349–64.

Bestall, J., Ahmed, N., Ahmedzai, S., Payne, S., Noble, B. and Clark, D. (2004) Access and referral to specialist palliative care. *International Journal of Palliative Nursing* 10(8), 381–89.

Bishop, F. and Yardley, L. (2004). Constructing agency in treatment decisions. *Health* 8(4), 465–82.

Bolletino, R. (2001). A model of spirituality for psychotherapy and other fields of mind–body medicine. *Advances in Mind–Body Medicine* 17(2), 90–107.

Bolton, S. (2001) Changing faces: Nurses as emotional jugglers. *Sociology of Health and Illness* 23(1), 85–100.

Booth, J. (1994) On the idea of the moral economy. *American Political Science Review* 88(3), 653–67.

Bradshaw. A. (1996) The spiritual dimension of hospice: The secularization of an ideal. *Social Science & Medicine* 43(3), 409–19.

Breitbart, W., Rosenfeld, B., Pessin, H., Kaim, M., Funesti-Esch, J. and Galietta, M. (2000) Depression, hopelessness and desire for death in terminally ill patients with cancer. *Journal of American Medical Association* 284(22), 2907–15. DOI: 10.1001/jama.284.22.2907.

Brenner, H. (2002). Long-term survival rates of cancer patients achieved by the end of the 20th century: a period analysis. *The Lancet* 360(9340), 1131–35.

Brickner, L., Scannell, K., Marquet, S. and Ackerson, L. (2004) Barriers to hospice care and referrals. *Journal of Palliative Medicine* 7(3), 411–18.

Broom, A. (2009a) "I'd forgotten about me in all of this": Discourses of self-healing, positivity and vulnerability in cancer patients' experiences of complementary and alternative medicine. *Journal of Sociology* 45(1), 71–87. DOI: 10.1177/1440783308099987.

Broom, A. (2009b). Intuition, subjectivity and *le bricoleur*: Cancer patients' accounts of negotiating a plurality of therapeutic options. *Qualitative Health Research* 19(8), 1050–59.

Broom, A. (2009c) The sociology of complementary and alternative medicine. In J. Germov (ed.) *Second Opinion*, 433–51. Melbourne: Oxford University Press.

Broom, A. (2012a) On euthanasia, resistance and redemption: The moralities and politics of a hospice. *Qualitative Health Research* 22(2), 226–37.

Broom, A. (2012b) Gender and end-of-life care. In Kuhlmann, E. and Annandale, E. (eds), *The Palgrave Handbook of Gender and Healthcare*. London: Palgrave Macmillan.

Broom, A. and Adams, J. (2010) The reconfiguration of expertise in oncology: The practice of prediction and articulation of indeterminacy in medical consultations. *Qualitative Health Research* 20(10), 1433–45. DOI: 10.1177/1049732310373042.

Broom, A. and Cavenagh, J. (2010) Moralities, masculinities and caring for the dying. *Social Science & Medicine* 71(5), 869–76. DOI: 10.1016/j.socscimed.2010.05.026.

Broom, A. and Cavenagh, J. (2011) On the meanings and experiences of living and dying in a hospice. *Health* 15(1), 96–111. DOI: 10.1177/1363459309360797.

Broom, A. and Doron, A. (2012) The rise of cancer in urban India: Cultural understandings, structural inequalities, and the emergence of the clinic. *Health* 16(3), 250–66.

Broom, A. and Doron, A. (2013) Traditional medicines, collective negotiation, and representations of risk in Indian cancer care. *Qualitative Health Research* 23(1), 54–65. DOI: 10.1177/1049732312462242.

Broom, A. and Kirby, E. (2013) The end of life and the family: Hospice patients' views on dying as relational. *Sociology of Health and Illness* 35(4), 499–513.

Broom, A. and Tovey, P. (2007a) Therapeutic Pluralism? Evidence, power and legitimacy in UK cancer services. *Sociology of Health and Illness* 29(3), 551–69.

Broom, A. and Tovey, P. (2007b) The dialectical tension between individuation and depersonalisation in cancer patients' mediation of complementary, alternative and biomedical cancer treatments. *Sociology* 41(6), 1021–39.

Broom, A. and Tovey, P. (2008) Exploring the temporal dimension in cancer patients' experiences of non-biomedical therapeutics. *Qualitative Health Research* 18(12), 1650–61. DOI: 10.1177/1049732308326511.

Broom, A. and Tovey, P. (2008) *Therapeutic Pluralism: Exploring the Experiences of Cancer Patients and Professionals*. Routledge: London and New York.

Broom, A. and Tovey, P. (eds.) (2009) *Men's Health: Body, Identity and Social Context*. Oxford: Wiley-Blackwell.

Broom, A., Doron, A. and Tovey, P. (2009) The inequalities of medical pluralism: Hierarchies of health, the politics of tradition and the economies of care in Indian oncology. *Social Science & Medicine* 69(5), 698–706.

Broom, A., Kirby, E., Good, P., Wootton, J. and Adams, J. (2013a) The art of letting go: Referral to palliative care and its discontents. *Social Science & Medicine* 78, 9–16. DOI: 10.1016/j.socscimed.2012.11.008.

Broom, A., Good, P., Kirby, E. and Lwin, Z. (2013b) Negotiating palliative care in the context of culturally and linguistically diverse patients. *Internal Medicine Journal* 43(9), 1043–46 DOI: 10.1111/imj.12244.

Broom, A., Kirby, E., Good, P., Wootton, J., Hardy, J., Yates, P. (2014) Negotiating futility, managing emotions: Nursing the transition to palliative care. *Qualitative Health Research.* DOI: 1049732314553123.

Broom, A., Kirby, E., Good, P., Wootton, J. and Adams, J. (2014b) The troubles of telling: Managing communication about the end of life. *Qualitative Health Research* 24(2), 151–62. DOI: 10.1177/1049732313519709.

Broom, A., Meurk, C., Adams, J. and Sibbritt, D (2014c) Networks of knowledge or just old wives' tales? A diary-based analysis of women's self-care practices and everyday lay expertise. *Health* 18(4), 335–51.

Broom, A., Kirby, E., Adams, J. and Refshuage, K. (2014c) On illegitimacy, suffering and recognition: A diary study of women living with chronic pain. *Sociology* DOI: 10.1177/0038038514551090.

Brown, C.G. (2009). *The Death of Christian Britain: Understanding Secularisation, 1800–2000.* Abingdon: Routledge.

Brown, R., Dunn, S., Byrnes, K., Morris, R., Heinrich, P. and Shaw, J. (2009) Doctors' stress responses and poor communication performance in simulated bad-news consultations. *Academic Medicine* 84(11), 1595–1602.

Burkitt, I. (1999). *Bodies of Thought: Embodiment, Identity and Modernity.* London: Sage.

Burt, R.A. (2002) The medical futility debate: Patient choice, physician obligation, and end-of-life care. *Journal of Palliative Medicine* 5(2), 249–54.

Campbell, T., Carey, E., Jackson, V., Saraiya, B., Yang, H., Back, A. and Arnold, R. (2010) Discussing prognosis: Balancing hope and realism. *The Cancer Journal* 16(5), 461–66.

Cannaerts, N., Dierckx de Casterlé, B. and Grypdonck, M. (2004) Palliative care, care for life: A study of the specificity of residential palliative care. *Qualitative Health Research* 14(6), 816–35.

Castleden, H., Crooks, V. A., Schuurman, N. and Hanlon, N. (2010) "It's not necessarily the distance on the map...": Using place as an analytic tool to elucidate geographic issues central to rural palliative care. *Health and Place* 16(2), 284–90.

Centers for Disease Control and Prevention (CDC). (2005) Annual smoking-attributable mortality, years of potential life lost, and productivity losses–United States, 1997–2001. *Morbidity and Mortality Weekly Report* 54(25), 625–8.

Chabner, B.A. and Roberts, T.G. (2005) Chemotherapy and the war on cancer. *Nature Reviews Cancer* 5(1), 65–72.

Chapple, A., Ziebland, S. and Hawton, K. (2015) Taboo and the different death? Perceptions of those bereaved by suicide or other traumatic death. Article first published online: 13 February 2015. DOI: 10.1111/1467-9566.12224.

Chapple, A., Ziebland, S. and McPherson, A. (2006) The specialist palliative care nurse: A qualitative study of the patients' perspective. *International Journal of Nursing Studies* 43(8), 1011–22.

Chattoo, S. and Ahmad, W. (2008) The moral economy of selfhood and caring. *Sociology of Health and Illness* 30(4), 550–64. DOI: 10.1111/j.1467-9566.2007.01072.x.

Christ, G. and Blacker, S. (2005) Improving interdisciplinary communication skills with families. *Journal of Palliative Medicine* 8(4), 855–56.

Christakis, N. (1999) *Death Foretold.* Chicago: University of Chicago Press.

Clark, C. (1990) Emotions and micropolitics in everyday life: Some patterns and paradoxes of "place". In T. Kemper (ed.), *Research Agendas in the Sociology of Emotions.* Albany: State University of New York Press, pp. 305–33.

Clark, D. (1993) *The Sociology of Death.* Oxford: Blackwell.

Clark, D. (2002) Between hope and acceptance: The medicalisation of dying. *British Medical Journal* 324(7342), 905–7. DOI: 10.1136/bmj.324.7342.905.

Clark, D. (2007) From margins to centre: A review of the history of palliative care in cancer. *Lancet Oncology* 8(5), 430–38. DOI: 10.1016/S1470-2045(07)70138-9.

Clark, D. and Seymour, J. (1999) *Reflections on Palliative Care: Sociological and Policy Perspectives.* London: Oxford University Press.

Clark, M., Rummans, T., Sloan, J., Jensen, A., Atherton, P., Frost, M., Richardson, J., Bostwick, J., Johnson, M., Hanson, J. and Brown, P. (2006) Quality of life of caregivers of patients with advanced-stage cancer, *American Journal of Hospice and Palliative Medicine* 23(3), 185–91.

Clayton, J., Butow, P., Arnold, R. and Tattersall, M. (2005) Discussing end-of-life issues with terminally ill cancer patients and their carers: A qualitative study. *Supportive Care in Cancer* 13(8), 589–99.

Cobb, M. (2001) *The Dying Soul: Spiritual Care at the End of Life.* Buckingham: Open University Press.

Costello, J. (2006) Dying well: nurses' experiences of 'good and bad' deaths in hospital. *Journal of Advanced Nursing* 54(5), 594–601.

Crocker, H. (2002) Methodological issues in male caregiver research. *Journal of Advanced Nursing* 40(6), 626–40.

Crossley, N. (1995) Merleau-Ponty, the elusive body and carnal sociology. *Body and Society* 1(1), 43–63.

Davis, K. (2013) *Reshaping the Female Body: The Dilemma of Cosmetic Surgery*. New York: Routledge.

Denier, Y., Dierckx de Casterlé, B., De Bal, N. and Gastmans, C. (2010) "It's intense, you know": Nurses' experiences in caring for patients requesting euthanasia. *Medicine, Health Care and Philosophy* 13(1), 41–8. DOI: 10.1007/s11019-009-9203-1.

Department of Health (2010) Introduction. The National Palliative Care Strategy – Supporting Australians to Live Well at the End of Life. Canberra: Commonwealth of Australia. http://www.health.gov.au/internet/publications/publishing.nsf/Content/ageing-npcs-2010-toc~ageing-npcs-2010-introduction.

De Raeve, L. (1997) Positive thinking and moral oppression in cancer care. *European Journal of Cancer Care* 6(4), 249–56.

Donchin, A. (2000) Autonomy, interdependence, and assisted suicide. *Bioethics* 14(3), 187–204. DOI: 10.1111/1467-8519.00190.

Doron, A. and Broom, A. (eds) (2011) *Health, Culture and Religion in South Asia: Critical Perspectives*. London and New York: Routledge.

Dowbiggin, I. (2002) *A Merciful End*. New York: Oxford University Press.

Du Boulay, S. and Rankin, M. (1984) *Cicely Saunders: Founder of the Modern Hospice Movement*. London: Hodder and Stoughton.

Edmondson, D., Park, C., Chaudoir, S. and Wortmann, J. (2008) Death without God: Religious struggle, death concerns, and depression in the terminally ill. *Psychological Science* 19(8), 754–8. DOI: 10.1111/j.1467-9280.2008.02152.x.

Eliott, J. and Olver, I. (2007) The implications of dying cancer patients' talk on cardiopulmonary resuscitation and do-not-resuscitate orders: A discursive analysis. *Qualitative Health Research* 17(4), 442–55. DOI: 10.1177/1049732307299198.

Eliott, J. and Olver, I. (2008) Dying cancer patients talk about euthanasia. *Social Science & Medicine* 67(4), 647–56. DOI: 10.1016/j.socscimed.2008.04.004.

Elsayem, A., Swint, K., Fisch, M.J., Palmer, J.L., Reddy, S., Walker, P., and Bruera, E. (2004) Palliative care inpatient service in a comprehensive cancer center: Clinical and financial outcomes. *Journal of Clinical Oncology* 22(10), 2008–14.

Emanuel, E.J. and Emanuel, L.L. (1994). The economics of dying: The illusion of cost savings at the end of life. *New England Journal of Medicine* 330(8), 540–44.

Emanuel, E.J., and Emanuel, L.L. (1998). The promise of a good death. *The Lancet* 351, SII21-SII29.

Emanuel, E., Fairclough, D., Daniels, E. and Clarridge, B. (1996) Euthanasia and physician-assisted suicide: Attitudes and experiences of oncology patients, oncologists, and the public. *Lancet* 347(9018), 1805–10. DOI: 10.1016/S0140-6736(96)91621-9.

Emslie, C., Browne, S., MacLeod, U., Rozmovits, L., Mitchell, E. and Ziebland, S. (2009) "Getting through" not "going under": A qualitative study of gender and spousal support after diagnosis with colorectal cancer. *Social Science & Medicine* 68(6), 1169–75.

Exley, C., and Allen, D. (2007) A critical examination of home care: end of life care as an illustrative case. *Social Science & Medicine* 65(11), 2317–2327. DOI: 10.1016/j.socscimed.2007.07.006.

Exley, C. and Letherby, G. (2001) Managing a disrupted lifecourse: Issues of identity and emotion work. *Health* 5(1), 112–32.

Exline, J.J. and Yali, A.M. (2000) Guilt, discord and alienation: The role of religious strain in depression and suicidality. *Journal of Clinical Psychology* 56(12), 1481–96. DOI: 10.1002/1097-4679.

Faunce, W.A. and Fulton, R.L. (1958) The sociology of death: A neglected area of research? *Social Forces* 36, 205–9.

Field, D. (1989) *Nursing the Dying.* London: Tavistock/Routledge.

Field, D., Hockey, J. and Small, N. (eds) (1997) *Death, Gender and Ethnicity.* London: Routledge.

Field, D., Dand, P., Ahmedzai, S. and Biswas, B. (1993) Lay carers of patients admitted to a hospice: How caring restricts their lives. *Health and Social Care* 1(3), 161–68.

Fillion, L., Tremblay, I., Truchon, M., Côté, D., Struthers, C.W. and Dupuis, R. (2007) Job satisfaction and emotional distress among nurses providing palliative care. *International Journal of Stress Management* 14(1), 1–25.

Fine, M. (2007) *A Caring Society? Care and the Dilemmas of Human Service in the Twenty-first Century.* Basingstoke: Palgrave Macmillan.

Fisher, L. and Lieberman, M. (1999) A longitudinal study of predictors of nursing home placement for patients with dementia. *The Gerontologist* 39(6), 677–86.

Foucault, M. (1977) *Discipline and Punish: The Birth of the Prison.* New York: Random House LLC.

Foucault, M. (1988) Technologies of the self. In L.H. Martin, H. Gutman and P.H. Hutton (eds) *Technologies of the Self: A Seminar with Michel Foucault.* Amherst: The University of Massachusetts Press.

Fox, J. (2006) "Notice how you feel": An alternative to detached concern among hospice volunteers. *Qualitative Health Research* 16(7), 944–61.

Fox, R.C. (1959) *Experiment Perilous.* Glencoe, IL: Free Press.

Fox, R.C. and Lief, H. (1963) Training for "detached concern". In Lief, H. (ed.) *The Psychological Basis of Medical Practice.* New York: Harper and Row.

Frank, A. (1991). *At the Will of the Body.* New York: Houghton Mifflin.

Frank, A. (1997) Illness as moral occasion: restoring agency to ill people. *Health* 1(2), 131–48. DOI: 10.1177/136345939700100201.

Frank A. (2005) The remission society. In P. Conrad (ed.) *The Sociology of Health and Illness*. New York: Worth Publishers, pp. 163–6.

Frank A. (2003) Survivorship as craft and conviction. *Qualitative Health Research* 13(2), 247–55.

Fraser N. (2000) Rethinking recognition. *New Left Review* 3(May-June), 107–20.

Freidson, E. (1988) *Profession of Medicine*. Chicago: University of Chicago Press.

Friedman, T., Harwood, K. and Shields, M. (2002) Barriers and enablers to hospice referrals. *Journal of Palliative Medicine* 5(1), 73–84.

Friedrichsen, M. and Strang, P. (2003) Doctors' strategies when breaking bad news to terminally ill patients. *Journal of Palliative Medicine* 6(4), 565–74.

Froggatt, K. (1997) Rites of passage and the hospice culture. *Mortality* 2(2), 123–36.

Froggatt, K. (1998) The place of metaphor and language in exploring nurses' emotional work. *Journal of Advanced Nursing* 28(2), 332–38.

Froggatt, K. (2001). Life and death in English nursing homes: sequestration or transition? *Ageing and Society* 21(3), 319–32.

Gaydos, H.L.B. (2004) The living end: Life journeys of hospice nurses. *Journal of Hospice and Palliative Nursing* 6(1), 17–26.

Giddens, A. (1991) *Modernity and Self-identity*. Stanford, CA: Stanford University Press.

Givens, J. and Mitchell, S. (2009) Concerns about end-of-life care and support for euthanasia. *Journal of Pain and Symptom Management* 38(2), 167–73. DOI: 0.1016/j.jpainsymman.2008.08.012.

Glaser, B. and Strauss, A. (1965) *Awareness of Dying*. Chicago: Aldine.

Glaser, B. and Strauss, A. (1968) *Time for Dying*. Chicago: Aldine.

Goldberg, J. (2010) Family carers in palliative care. *Journal of Palliative Medicine* 13(3), 339–40.

Good, M-J., Good, B., Schaffer, C. and Lind, S. 1990. American oncology and the discourse on hope. *Culture, Medicine and Psychiatry* 14(1), 59–79.

Gordon, S. (1990). Social structural effects on emotion. In T. Kemper (ed.), *Research Agendas in the Sociology of Emotions*. Albany: State University of New York Press, pp. 145–79.

Gott, M., Small, N., Barnes, S., Payne, S. and Seamark, D. (2008) Older people's views of a good death in heart failure. *Social Science & Medicine* 67(7), 1113–21. DOI: 10.1016/j.socscimed.2008.05.024.

Gott, M., Ingleton, C., Bennett, M. I. and Gardiner, C. (2011) Transitions to palliative care in acute hospitals in England: Qualitative study. *BMJ Supportive and Palliative Care* 1(1), 42–8.

Graham, R. (2006) Lacking compassion: Sociological analyses of the medical profession. *Social Theory and Health* 4(1), 43–63.

Grande, G., Addington-Hall, J. and Todd, C. (1998) Place of death and access to home care services. *Social Science & Medicine* 47(5), 565–79.

Grande, G., Todd, C. and Barclays, S. (1997). Support needs in the last year of life: Patient and carer dilemmas. *Palliative Medicine* 11(3), 202–8.

Grande, G., Stajduhar, K., Aoun, S., Toye, C., Funk, L., Addington-Hall, J.,Payne, S., Todd, C. (2009) Supporting lay carers in end of life care. *Palliative Medicine* 23(4), 339–44.

Gray, B. (2010) Emotional labour, gender and professional stereotypes of emotional and physical contact, and personal perspectives on the emotional labour of nursing. *Journal of Gender Studies* 19(4), 349–60.

Gray, R. and Doan, B. 1990. Heroic self-healing and cancer: Clinical issues for the health professions. *Journal of Palliative Care* 6(1), 32–41.

Gross, N. (2005) The detraditionalization of intimacy reconsidered. *Sociological Theory* 23(3), 286–311.

Gysels, M., Shipman, C. and Higginson, I. (2008) Is the qualitative research interview an acceptable medium for research with palliative care patients and carers? *BMC Medical Ethics* 9(7). DOI: http://dx.doi.org/10.1136/bmj.b4122.

Hagerty, R., Butow, P., Ellis, P., Lobb, E., Pendlebury, S., Leighl, N., MacLeod, C. and Tattersall, M. (2005) Communicating with realism and hope. *Journal of Clinical Oncology* 23(6), 1278–88.

Hales, S., Zimmermann, C. and Rodin, G. (2008) The quality of dying and death. *Archives of Internal Medicine* 168(9), 912–18.

Hallam, E., Hockey, J. and Howarth, G. (1999) *Beyond the Body. Death and Social Identity.* London: Routledge.

Hanratty, B., Lowson, E., Holmes, L., Grande, G., Jacoby, A., Payne, S., Whitehead, M. (2012) Breaking bad news sensitively: What is important to patients in their last year of life? *BMJ Supportive and Palliative Care* 2(1), 24–8.

Harding, R. and Higginson, I. (2003) What is the best way to help caregivers in cancer and palliative care? *Palliative Medicine* 17(1), 63–74.

Hardy, J., Maresco-Pennisi, D., Gilshenan, K. and Yates, P. (2008) Barriers to the best care of the dying in Queensland, Australia. *Journal of Palliative Medicine* 11(10), 1330–35.

Hart, B., Sainsbury, P. and Short, S. (1998) Whose dying? A sociological critique of the "good death". *Mortality* 3(1), 65–77.

Hayley, D., Muir, J., Stocking, C., Hougham, G. and Sachs, G. (2001). Not ready for hospice. *American Journal of Hospice and Palliative Care* 18(6), 377–82.

Heedman P-A. and Starkhammar, H. (2002) Patterns of referral to a palliative care unit. *Journal of Palliative Medicine* 5(1), 101–6.

Henderson, A. (2001) Emotional labor and nursing: An under-appreciated aspect of caring work. *Nursing Inquiry* 8(2), 130–38.

Hewitt M., Greenfield, S. and Stovall, E.(eds) (2005) *From Cancer Patient to Cancer Survivor: Lost in Transition.* Washington: National Academic Press.

Hibbert, D., Hanratty, B., May, C., Mair, F., Litva, A. and Capewell, S. (2003) Negotiating palliative care expertise in the medical world. *Social Science & Medicine* 57(2), 277–88.

Higginson, I. and Sen-Gupta, G. (2000) Place of care in advanced cancer. *Journal of Palliative Medicine* 3(3), 287–300.

Hobbes, T. (1670) *Leviathan.* Amstelodami: Joannem Blaev.

Hochschild, A.R. (1979) Emotion work, feeling rules, and social structure. *American Journal of Sociology* 85(3), 551–75.

Hochschild, A. (1983) *The Managed Heart.* Berkeley: University of California Press.

Hockey, J.L. (1990) *Experiences of Death: An Anthropological Account.* Edinburgh: Edinburgh University Press.

Hockey, J.L., Komaromy, C. and Woodthorpe, K. (2010) *The Matter of Death: Space, Place and Materiality.* Basingstoke: Palgrave Macmillan.

House, J.S. (2002). Understanding social factors and inequalities in health: 20th century progress and 21st century prospects. *Journal of Health and Social Behavior* 43(2), 125–42.

Howarth, G. (2007a) 'Dying: Institutionalization and Medicalization.' In G. Howarth (ed.), *Death and Dying: A Sociological Introduction.* Cambridge: Polity Press, pp. 115–31.

Howarth, G. (2007b) *Death and Dying: A Sociological Introduction.* Cambridge: Polity Press.

Howarth, G. (2007c) Whatever happened to social class? An examination of the neglect of working class cultures in the sociology of death. *Health Sociology Review* 16(5), 425–35.

Howson, A. and Inglis, D. (2001) The body in sociology: Tensions inside and outside sociological thought. *The Sociological Review* 49(3), 297–317.

Hudson, P., Aranda, S. and Kristjanson, L. (2004) Meeting the supportive needs of family caregivers in palliative care. *Journal of Palliative Medicine* 7(1), 19–25.

Hudson, P. and Payne, S. (2011) Family caregivers and palliative care. *Journal of Palliative Medicine* 14(7), 864–69.

Hudson, P.L., Remedios, C. and Thomas, K. (2010) A systematic review of psychosocial interventions for family carers of palliative care patients. *BMC Palliative Care* 9(17), 1–6.

Hughes, B. and Paterson, K. (1997) The social model of disability and the disappearing body: Towards a sociology of impairment. *Disability and Society* 12(3), 325–40.

Illick, I. (1976) *Limits to Medicine.* London: Marion Boyers.

James, J. (1989) Emotional labour: Skill and work in the social regulation of feelings. *Sociological Review* 37(1), 15–42.

James, N. and Field, D. (1992) The routinization of hospice: Charisma and bureaucratization. *Social Science & Medicine* 34(12), 1363–75. DOI: 10.1016/0277-9536(92)90145-G.

Jamieson, L. (1998) *Intimacy*. Cambridge: Polity Press.

Johansen, S., Holen, J., Kaasa, S., Loge, H. and Materstvedt, L. (2005) Attitudes towards, and wishes for, euthanasia in advanced cancer patients at a palliative care unit. *Palliative Medicine* 19(6), 454–60. DOI: 10.1191/0269216305pm1048oa.

Johnson, B., and Clarke, J.M. (2003) Collecting Sensitive Data: The Impact on Researchers. *Qualitative Health Research* 13(3), 421–34. DOI: 10.1177/1049732302250340.

Johnson, C., Girgis, A., Paul, C. and Currow, D. (2008) Cancer specialists' palliative care referral practices and perceptions. *Palliative Medicine* 22(1), 51–7.

Johnson, C., Paul, C., Girgis, A., Adams, J. and Currow, D.C. (2011) Australian general practitioners' and oncology specialists' perceptions of barriers and facilitators of access to specialist palliative care services. *Journal of Palliative Medicine* 14(4), 429–35.

Kaiser, K. (2008) The meaning of the survivor identity for women with breast cancer. *Social Science & Medicine* 67(1), 79–87.

Karp, D. and Tanarugsachock, V. (2000) Mental illness, caregiving, and emotion management. *Qualitative Health Research* 10(1), 6–25.

Kellehear, A. (1984) Are we a death denying society? A sociological review. *Social Science & Medicine* 18(9), 713–23.

Kellehear, A. (1990) *Dying of Cancer*. Melbourne: Harwood.

Kellehear, A. (2007) *A Social History of Dying*. Cambridge: Cambridge University Press.

Kellehear, A. (2008) Dying as a social relationship. *Social Science & Medicine* 66(7), 1533–44. DOI: 10.1016/j.socscimed.2007.12.023.

Kellehear, A. (ed.) (2009) *The Study of Dying*. Cambridge: Cambridge University Press.

Kelly, M.P. and Field, D. (1996) Medical sociology, chronic illness and the body. *Sociology of Health and Illness* 18(2), 241–57.

Kelly, B., Burnett, P., Pelusi, D., Badger, S., Varghese, F. and Robertson, M. (2002) Terminally ill cancer patients› wish to hasten death. *Palliative Medicine* 16(4), 339–45. DOI: 10.1191/0269216302pm538oa.

Kendall, M., Harris, F., Boyd, K., Sheikh, A., Murray, S., Brown, D., Mallinson, I., Kearney, N. and Worth, A. (2007) Key challenges and ways forward in researching the "good death". *British Medical Journal* 334(7592), 521–4.

King, D. and Quill, T. (2006) Working with families in palliative care: One size does not fit all. *Journal of Palliative Medicine* 9(3), 704–15.

Kirby, E., Broom, A., Good, P., Wootton, J. and Adams, J. (2014a) Families and the transition to specialist palliative care. *Mortality*. DOI: http://dx.doi.org/10.1080/13576275.2014.916258.

Kirby, E., Broom, A., Good, P. (2014b) The role and significance of nurses in managing transitions to palliative care: A qualitative study. *British Medical Journal Open* 4(9), DOI: 10.1136/bmjopen-2014-006026.

Kirsi, T., Hervonen, A. and Jylha, M. (2004) Always one step behind: Husbands' narratives about taking care of their demented wives. *Health* 8(2), 159–81.

Kissane, D (2009) Beyond the psychotherapy and survival debate. *Psycho-Oncology* 18(1), 1–5.

Kramer, B., Boelk, A. and Auer, C. (2006) Family conflict at the end of life. *Journal of Palliative Medicine* 9(3), 791–801.

Kristeva, J. (1982) *Powers of Horror*. New York: Columbia University Press.

Kristjanson, L. (2005) Directions in palliative care nursing research: impeccable care, timing and complexity. *Canadian Journal of Nursing Research* 37(2), 13–20.

Kristjanson, L. and Aoun, S. (2004) Palliative care for families. *Canadian Journal of Psychiatry* 49(6), 359–65.

Kubler-Ross, E. (1969) *On Death and Dying*. New York: Macmillan.

Kuuppelomäki, M. (2000). Attitudes of cancer patients, their family members and health professionals toward active euthanasia. *European Journal of Cancer Care* 9(1), 16–21.

Laslett, P. (1991) *A Fresh Map of Life: The Emergence of the Third Age*. Cambridge, MA: Harvard University Press.

Lawton, J. (1998) Contemporary hospice care: The sequestration of the unbounded body and "dirty dying". *Sociology of Health and Illness* 20(2), 121–43.

Lawton, J. (2000) *The Dying Process*. Routledge.

Lee, R. (2008) Modernity, Mortality and Re-Enchantment: The Death Taboo Revisited. *Sociology* 42(4), 745–59. DOI: 10.1177/0038038508091626.

Li, S. (2004) "Symbiotic niceness": Constructing a therapeutic relationship in psychosocial palliative care. *Social Science & Medicine* 58(12), 2571–83.

Li, S. and Arber, A. (2006) The construction of troubled and credible patients: A study of emotion talk in palliative care settings. *Qualitative Health Research* 16, 27–46.

Liamputtong, P. (2006) *Researching the Vulnerable: A Guide to Sensitive Research Methods*. London: SAGE.

Little, M., Jordens, C., Paul, K., Montgomery, K. and Philipson, B. (1998) Liminality: A major category of the experience of cancer illness. *Social Science & Medicine* 47(10), 1485–94.

Lloyd-Williams, M., Wright, M., Cobb, M. and Shiels, C. (2004) A prospective study of the roles, responsibilities and stresses of chaplains working within a hospice. *Palliative Medicine* 18(7), 638–45. DOI: 10.1191/0269216304pm929oa.

Lofland, L.H. (ed.) (1976) *Toward a Sociology of Death and Dying* (Vol. 28). Beverly Hills, CA: Sage.

Lofmark, R., Nilstun, T. and Bolmsjo, I. (2005) From cure to palliation: Staff communication, documentation, and transfer of patient. *Journal of Palliative Medicine* 8(6), 1105–9.

Lubitz, J., Cai, L., Kramarow, E., and Lentzner, H. (2003). Health, life expectancy, and health care spending among the elderly. *New England Journal of Medicine* 349(11), 1048–55.

Lupton, D. (1997) Doctors on the medical profession. *Sociology of Health and Illness* 19(4), 480–97.

MacArtney, J., Broom, A., Kirby, E., Good, P., Wootton, J., Adams, J. (2014) On resilience and acceptance in the transition to palliative care at the end of life. *Health*, 1–17. DOI: 10.1177/1363459314545696.

McClean, S. (2005) "The illness is part of the person": Discourses of blame, individual responsibility and individuation at a centre for spiritual healing in the North of England. *Sociology of Health and Illness* 27(5), 628–48.

McLennon, S., Habermann, B. and Davis, L. (2010) Deciding to institutionalize: Why do family members cease caregiving at home? *Journal of Neuroscience Nurs*ing 42(2), 95–103.

McMillan, S., Small, B., Weitzner, M., Schonwetter, R., Tittle, M., Moody, L. and Haley, W. (2006) Impact of coping skills intervention with family caregivers of hospice patients with cancer. *Cancer* 106(1), 214–22.

McNamara, B. (2001) *Fragile Lives: Death, Dying and Care*. Buckingham: Open University Press.

McNamara, B. (2004) Good enough death: Autonomy and choice in Australian palliative care. *Social Science & Medicine* 58(5), 929–38.

McNamara, B., Waddell, C. and Colvin, M. (1994) The institutionalisation of the good death. *Social Science & Medicine* 39(11), 1501–8.

McNamara, B., Waddell, C. and Colvin, M. (1995) Threats to the good death: The cultural context of stress and coping among hospice nurses. *Sociology of Health and Illness* 17(2), 222–41.

McPherson, C., Wilson, K. and Murray, M. (2007) Feeling like a burden: Exploring the perspectives of patients at the end of life. *Social Science & Medicine* 64(2), 417–27. DOI: 10.1016/j.socscimed.2006.09.013.

McQueen, A.C. (2004) Emotional intelligence in nursing work. *Journal of Advanced Nursing* 47(1), 101–8.

McSteen, K. and Peden-McAlpine, C. (2006) The role of the nurse as advocate in ethically difficult care situations with dying patients. *Journal of Hospice and Palliative Nursing* 8(5), 259–69.

Mak, Y. and Elwyn, G. (2005) Voices of the terminally ill: Uncovering the meaning of desire for euthanasia. *Palliative Medicine* 19(4), 343–50. DOI: 10.1191/0269216305pm1019oa.

Mak, Y., Elwyn, G. and Finlay, I.G. (2003) Patients' voices are needed in debates on euthanasia. *British Medical Journal* 327(7408), 213–15. DOI: 10.1136/bmj.327.7408.213.

May, W. (1991) *The Patient's Ordeal.* Bloomington: Indiana University Press.

Maynard, D. (1996) On "realization" in everyday life: The forecasting of bad news as a social relation. *American Sociological Review* 61(1), 109–31.

Mellor, P. and Shilling, C. (1993) Modernity, self identity and the sequestration of death. *Sociology* 27(3), 411–31.

Melvin, S., and Oldham, L. (2009). When to refer patients to palliative care: triggers, traps and timely referrals. *Journal of Hospice and Palliative Nursing* 11(5), 291–301.

Merleau-Ponty, M. (1996). *Phenomenology of Perception.* Motilal Banarsidass Publishers.

Meyer, M. (1995) Dignity, death and modern virtue. *American Philosophical Quarterly* 32, 45–56.

Miller, K.L., Reeves, S., Zwarenstein, M., Beales, J.D., Kenaszchuk, C. and Conn, L.G. (2008) Nursing emotion work and inter-professional collaboration in general internal medicine wards: A qualitative study. *Journal of Advanced Nursing* 64(4), 332–43.

Miracle, V. A. (2008) The life and impact of Florence Nightingale. *Dimensions of Critical Care Nursing* 27(1), 21–3.

Mitchell, G. (2011) Palliative Care in Australia. *The Ochsner Journal* 11(4), 334–37.

Mohammed, S. and Peter, E. (2009) Rituals, death and the moral practice of medical futility. *Nursing Ethics* 16(3), 292–302. DOI: 10.1177/0969733009102691.

Mok, E. and Chiu, P.C. (2004) Nurse–patient relationships in palliative care. *Journal of Advanced Nursing* 48(5), 475–83.

Morgan, D. (1993). "You too can have a body like mine": reflections on the male body and masculinities. In Scott, S. and Morgan, D. (eds), *Body Matters: Essays on the Sociology of the Body.* London: Falmer Press, pp. 69–88.

Morita, T., Akechi, T., Ikenaga, M., Kizawa, Y., Kohara, H., Mukaiyama, T., Nakaho, T., Nakashima, N., Shima, Y., Matsubara, T., Fujimori, M. and Uchitomi, Y. (2004) Communication about the ending of anticancer treatment and transition to palliative care. *Annals of Oncology* 15(10), 1551–7.

Morita, T., Miyashita, M., Kimura, R., Adachi, I. and Shima, Y. (2004) Emotional burden of nurses in palliative sedation therapy. *Palliative Medicine* 18(6), 550–57.

Morris, S.M. and Thomas, C. (2007) Placing the dying body: Emotional, situational and embodied factors in preferences for place of final care and death in cancer. In Davidson, J., Bondi, L. and Smith, M. (eds.) *Emotional Geographies*, pp. 19–31.

Morrison, R.S., Penrod, J.D., Cassel, J.B., Caust-Ellenbogen, M., Litke, A., Spragens, L., and Meier, D.E. (2008) Cost savings associated with US hospital palliative care consultation programs. *Archives of Internal Medicine* 168(16), 1783–90.

Murray, S. (2007) Care and the self: Biotechnology, reproduction, and the good life. *Philosophy, Ethics, and Humanities in Medicine* 2(6). DOI: 10.1186/1747-5341-2-6.

Murray, M., O'Connor, A., Fiset, V. and Viola, R. (2003) Women's decision making needs regarding place of care at end of life. *Journal of Palliative Care* 19(3), 176–84.

Najjar, N., Davis, L., Beck-Coon, K. and Carney Doebbeling, C. (2009) Compassion fatigue: A review of the research to date and relevance to cancer-care providers. *Journal of Health Psychology* 14(2), 267–77.

National Institutes of Health (NIH) (2011) Global Health and Aging. Access online at: http://www.nia.nih.gov/sites/default/files/global_health_and_aging.pdf [Accessed: 10/11/2014].

Navona, L. and Morag, A. (2004) Liminality as biographical disruption: Unclassifiability following hormonal therapy for advanced prostate cancer. *Social Science & Medicine* 58(11), 2337–47.

Nebel, S. (2011) Facing death together: Exploring the conceptualizations of hospice patients and family as a single unit of care, *Journal of Hospice and Palliative Nursing* 13(6), 419–25.

Nettleton, S. (2010) The Sociology of the Body. In Cockerham, W. (ed.) *The New Blackwell Companion to Medical Sociology*. London: Wiley-Blackwell, pp. 47–68.

Nettleton, S., Burrows, R. and Watt, I. (2008) How do you feel doctor? An analysis of emotional aspects of routine professional medical work. *Social Theory and Health* 6(1), 18–36.

Nissim, R., Gagliese, L. and Rodin, G. (2009) The desire for hastened death in individuals with advanced cancer: A longitudinal qualitative study. *Social Science & Medicine* 69(2), 165–71. DOI: 10.1016/j.socscimed.2009.04.021.

Noel-Miller, C. (2010) Spousal loss, children, and the risk of nursing home admission. *The Journal of Gerontology* 65B(3), 370–80.

Oliviere, D., Monroe, B. and Payne, S. (eds) (2011) *Death, Dying and Social Differences*. 2nd edn. Oxford: Oxford University Press.

Olson R. (2011) Managing hope, denial or temporal anomie? Informal cancer carers' accounts of spouses' cancer diagnoses. *Social Science & Medicine* 73(6), 904–11.

Parkinson, L., Rainbird, K., Kerridge, I., Carter, G., Cavenagh, J., McPhee, J., Ravenscroft, P. (2005) Cancer patients' attitudes towards euthanasia and physician-assisted suicide. *Journal of Bioethical Inquiry* 2(2), 82–89. DOI: 10.1007/BF02448847.

Parry, J. (1982) Sacrificial death and the necrophagous ascetic. In M. Bloch and J. Parry (eds) *Death and the Regeneration of Life*. Cambridge: Cambridge University Press.

Parry, J. (1994) *Death in Banaras*. Cambridge: Cambridge University Press.

Parsons, K. (1997) The male experience of caregiving for a family member with Alzheimer's disease. *Qualitative Health Research* 7(3), 391–407.

Payne, S., Langley-Evans, A. and Hillier, R. (1996) Perceptions of a 'good' death: A comparative study of the views of hospice staff and patients. *Palliative Medicine* 10(4), 307–12. DOI: 10.1177/026921639601000406.

Pargament, K.I., Koenig, H.G., Tarakeshwar, N. and Hahn, J. (2004) Religious coping methods as predictors of psychological, physical and spiritual outcomes among medically ill elderly patients. *Journal of Health Psychology* 9(6), 713–30. DOI: 10.1177/1359105304045366.

Petersen, A., Davis, M., Fraser, S., and Lindsay, J. (2010). Healthy living and citizenship: an overview. *Critical Public Health* 20(4), 391–400.

Phillips, S. (1996) Labouring the emotions: Expanding the remit of nursing work? *Journal of Advanced Nursing* 24(1), 139–43.

Phillips, J. and Currow, D. (2010) Cancer as a chronic disease. *Collegian* 17, 47–50.

Powell, A.E. and Davies, H.T. (2012) The struggle to improve patient care in the face of professional boundaries. *Social Science & Medicine* 75(5), 807–14.

Price, A. and Hotopf, M. (2009) The treatment of depression in patients with advanced cancer undergoing palliative care. *Current Opinion in Supportive and Palliative Care* 3(1), 61–6.

Prior, L. (1989) *The Social Organisation of Death*. London: Macmillan.

Ptacek, J. and Eberhardt, T. (1996) Breaking bad news: A review of the literature. *Journal of the American Medical Association* 276(6), 496–502.

Quill, T., Arnold, R. and Back, A. (2009) Discussing treatment preferences with patients who want "everything". *Annals of Internal Medicine* 151, 345–49.

Redinbaugh, E., Baum, A., Tarbell, S. and Arnold, R. (2003) End-of-life caregiving: What helps family caregivers cope? *Journal of Palliative Medicine* 6(6), 901–9.

Rietjens, J., Hauser, J. van der Heide, A. and Emanuel, L. (2007) Having a difficult time leaving: Experiences and attitudes of nurses with palliative sedation. *Palliative Medicine* 21(7), 643–49. DOI: 10.1177/0269216307081186.

Riley, J. (1983) Dying and the meanings of death: Sociological inquiries. *Annual Review of Sociology* 9, 191–216.

Rittenberg, C. (1995) Positive thinking: An unfair burden for cancer patients? *Supportive Care in Cancer* 3: 37–9.

Ronaldson, S. and Devery, K. (2001) The experience of transition to palliative care services: Perspectives of patients and nurses. *International Journal of Palliative Nursing* 7(4), 171–7.

Rose, N. (1999) *Governing the Soul*. London: Free Association Books.

Rose, N. (2001) The politics of life itself. *Culture, Theory and Society* 18(6), 1–30.

Rousseau, J. (1973) *The Social Contract* [translation and introduction by G.D.H. Cole]. London: Dent and Sons.

Rousseau, P. (2003). Death denial. *Journal of Clinical Oncology* 21(9 Suppl.), 52–3.

Rozmovits, L. and Ziebland, S. (2004) Expressions of loss of adulthood in the narratives of people with colorectal cancer. *Qualitative Health Research* 14(2), 187–203.

Sacks, J. and Nelson, J (2007) A theory of nonphysical suffering and trust in hospice patients. *Qualitative Health Research* 17(5), 675–89.

Salander, P. (2002) Bad news from the patient's perspective. *Social Science & Medicine* 55(5), 721–32.

Salhani, D. and Coulter, I. (2009) The politics of inter-professional working and the struggle for professional autonomy in nursing. *Social Science & Medicine* 68(7), 1221–8.

Sanders, T. and Harrison, S. (2008) Professional legitimacy claims in the multidisciplinary workplace. *Sociology of Health and Illness* 30(2), 289–308.

Sandgren, A., Thulesius, H., Fridlund, B. and Petersson, K. (2006) Striving for emotional survival in palliative cancer nursing. *Qualitative Health Research* 16(1), 79–96.

Saunders, C. (2000) The evolution of palliative care. *Patient Education and Counseling* 41(1), 7–13.

Sarenmalm, E., Thorén-Jönsson, A., Gaston-Johansson, F. and Öhlén, J. (2009) Making sense of living under the shadow of death: Adjusting to a recurrent breast cancer illness. *Qualitative Health Research* 19(8), 1116–30.

Sayer, A. (2005) Class, moral worth and recognition. *Sociology* 39(5), 947–63 DOI: 10.1177/0038038505058376.

Sayer, D. (2010) Who's afraid of the dead? Archaeology, modernity and the death taboo. *World Archaeology* 42(3), 481–91.

Schofield, P., Carey, M., Love, A., Nehill, C. and Wein, S. (2006) "Would you like to talk about your future treatment options?": Discussing the transition from curative cancer treatment to palliative care. *Palliative Medicine* 20(4), 397–406.

Schulman-Green, D., Mccorkle, R., Curry, L., Cherlin, E., Johnson-Hurzeler, R. and Bradley, E. (2004) At the crossroads: Making the transition to hospice. *Palliative and Supportive Care* 2(4), 351–60.

Scott, S. and Morgan, D. (eds) (1993) *Body Matters: Essays on the Sociology of the Body*. London: Falmer Press.

Seale, C. (1995). Heroic death. *Sociology* 29(4), 597–613.

Seale, C. (1998a) *Constructing Death: The Sociology of Dying and Bereavement.* Cambridge: Cambridge University Press.

Seale, C. (1998b) Social and ethical aspects of euthanasia: A review. *Progress in Palliative Care* 5(4), 141–6.

Seale, C. (2001) Sporting cancer: Struggle language in news reports of people with cancer. *Sociology of Health and Illness* 23(3), 308–29. DOI: 10.1111/1467-9566.00254.

Seale, C. (2002) Cancer heroics. *Sociology* 36(1), 107–26.

Seale, C. and Addington-Hall, J. (1994) Euthanasia: Why people want to die earlier. *Social Science & Medicine* 39(5), 647–54. DOI: 10.1016/0277-9536(94)90021-3.

Sepúlveda, C., Marlin, A., Yoshida, T., and Ullrich, A. (2002). Palliative Care: the World Health Organization's Global Perspective. *Journal of Pain and Symptom Management* 24(2), 91–6.

Sered, S., and Agigian, A. (2008). Holistic sickening: breast cancer and the discursive worlds of complementary and alternative practitioners. *Sociology of Health and Illness* 30(4), 616–31.

Seymour, J., Payne, S., Chapman, A., and Holloway, M. (2007) Hospice or home? Expectations of end-of-life care among white and Chinese older people in the UK. *Sociology of Health and Illness* 29(6), 872–90. DOI: 10.1111/j.1467-9566.2007.01045.x.

Shilling, C. (1993) *The Body and Social Theory*. London: Sage.

Shilling, C. (2007) Sociology and the body: Classical traditions and new agendas. *The Sociological Review* 55(s1), 1–18.

Shilling, C. (2012) *The Body and Social Theory*, 3rd edn. London Sage.

Shilling, C. and Mellor, P.A. (1996) Embodiment, structuration theory and modernity: Mind/body dualism and the repression of sensuality. *Body and Society* 2(4), 1–15.

Silverstein, M. and Giarrusso, R. (2010) Ageing and family life: A decade review, *Journal of Marriage and Family* 72(5), 1039–58.

Sivaramakrishnan, K. (2005) Moral economies, state spaces, and categorical violence. *American Anthropologist* 107(3), 321–402. DOI: 10.1525/aa.2005.107.3.321.

Skilbeck, J. and Payne, S. (2003) Emotional support and the role of clinical nurse specialists in palliative care. *Journal of Advanced Nursing* 43(5), 521–30.

Smart, C. (2007) *Personal Life: New Directions in Sociological Thinking*. Cambridge: Polity Press.

Smith, R. (2000). A good death. *British Medical Journal* 320(7228), 129–30.

Smith, T.J., Coyne, P., Cassel, B., Penberthy, L., Hopson, A., and Hager, M.A. (2003). A high-volume specialist palliative care unit and team may reduce in-hospital end-of-life care costs. *Journal of Palliative Medicine* 6(5), 699–705.

Smith, T., Dow, L., Virago, E., Khatcheressian, J., Lyckholm, L. and Matsuyama, R. (2010) Giving honest information to patients with advanced cancer maintains hope. *Oncology* 24(6), 521–5.

Smith, C., Nelson J., Berman A., Powell, C., Fleischmanm, J., Salazar-Schicchi and Wisnivesky, J. (2012) Lung cancer physicians' referral practices for palliative care consultation. *Annals of Oncology* 23(2), 382–87.

Sointu, E. 2006a. Healing bodies, feeling bodies. *Social Theory and Health* 4(3), 203–20.

Sointu, E. 2006b. Recognition and the creation of wellbeing. *Sociology* 40(3), 493–510.

Sointu, E. 2006c. The search for wellbeing in alternative and complementary health practices. *Sociology of Health and Illness* 28(3), 330–49.

Somerville, M. (2003) "Death talk": Debating euthanasia and physician-assisted suicide in Australia. *Medical Journal of Australia* 178(4), 171–4.

Sontag, S. (1991) *Illness as Metaphor and AIDS and its Metaphors*. Harmondsworth: Penguin Books.

Stacey, J. (1997) *Teratologies: A Cultural Study of Cancer*. London: Routledge.

Stajduhar, K., Funk, L., Jakobsson, E. and Ohlen, J. (2010) A critical analysis of health promotion and 'empowerment' in the context of palliative family care-giving. *Nursing Inquiry* 17(3), 221–30.

Stanley, L., and Wise, S. (2011). The Domestication of Death: The Sequestration Thesis and Domestic Figuration. *Sociology* 45(6), 947–62.

Stein, L.I. (1967). The doctor-nurse game. *Archives of General Psychiatry*, 16(6), 699.

Strauss, A.L. (1970) *Anguish: The Case History of a Dying Trajectory*. San Francisco: California Sociology Press.

Strauss, A.L. (1978) *Negotiations: Varieties, Contexts, Processes and Social Order*. London: Jossey-Bass.

Strauss, A., Schatzmann, L., Ehrlich, D., Bucher, R., and Sabshin, M. (1963). The hospital and its negotiated order. In Freidson, E. (ed.) *The Hospital in Modern Society*. New York: Free Press of Glencoe, pp. 147–69.

Strauss, A., Fagerhaugh, S., Suczek, B. and Wiener, C. (1982) Sentimental work in the technologized hospital. *Sociology of Health and Illness* 4(3), 254–78.

Steinhauser, K.E., Clipp, E.C., McNeilly, M., Christakis, N. A., McIntyre, L.M., and Tulsky, J.A. (2000) In search of a good death: observations of patients, families, and providers. *Annals of Internal Medicine* 132(10), 825–32.

Stenberg U., Ruland, C. M., and Miaskowski, C. (2010) Review of the literature on the effects of caring for a patient with cancer. *Psycho-Oncology* 19(10), 1013–25. DOI: 10.1002/pon.1670.

Strong, B., DeVault, C. and Cohen, T. (2010) *The Marriage and Family Experience*. Belmont, CA: Wadsworth.

Sulmasy, D.P. (2006) Spiritual issues in the care of dying patients. *Journal of the American Medical Association* 296(11), 1385–92. DOI: 10.1001/jama.296.11.1385.

Svensson, R. (1996) The interplay between doctors and nurses: A negotiated order perspective. *Sociology of Health and Illness* 18(3), 379–98.

Swetenham, K., Hegarty, M., Breaden, K. and Grbich, C. (2011) Refractory suffering. *Palliat Support Care* 9(1), 55–62.

Sykes, N. and Thorns, A. (2003) The use of opioids and sedatives at the end of life. *The Lancet Oncology* 4(5), 312–18.

Temel, J., Greer, J., Muzikansky, A., Gallagher, E., Admane, S., Jackson, V., Lynch, T. (2010) Early palliative care for patients with metastatic Non-Small-Cell lung cancer. *The New England Journal of Medicine* 363(8), 733–42.

The, A., Hak, T., Koeter, G. and van Der Wal, G. (2000) Collusion in doctor patient communication about imminent death: An ethnographic study. *British Medical Journal* 321(7273), 1376–81.

Theodosius, C. (2006) Recovering emotion from emotion management. *Sociology* 40(5), 893–910.

Thomas, C. (1993) Deconstructing concepts of care. *Sociology* 27(4), 649–69.

Thomas, C., Morris, S. and Harman, J. (2002) Companions through cancer: The care given by informal carers in cancer contexts. *Social Science & Medicine* 54(4), 529–44.

Thomas, C., Morris, S. and Clark, D. (2004) Place of death: Preferences among cancer patients and their carers. *Social Science & Medicine* 58(12), 2431–44.

Thorne, S., Hislop, T., Kuo, M. and Armstrong, E. (2006) Hope and probability. *Qualitative Health Research* 16(3), 318–36.

Tritter, J. and Calnan, M. (2002) Cancer as a chronic illness? *European Journal of Cancer Care* 11(3), 161–5.

Tronto, J. (1993) *Moral Boundaries: A Political Argument for an Ethic of Care*. New York: Routledge.

Tullis, J.A. (2012) Personhood and communication at the end of life. *Journal of Medicine and the Person* 10(3), 103–13.

Turner, B. S. (1984) *The Body and Society*. Oxford: Blackwell.

Turner, B.S. (1987) The Rationalization of the Body: Reflections on Modernity and Discipline in Whimster, S. and Lash, S. (eds.) *Max Weber, Rationality and Modernity*. London: Allen and Unwin, pp. 222–41.

Turner, B. S. (2011). *Religion and Modern Society: Citizenship, Secularisation and the State*. Cambridge: Cambridge University Press.

VandeKieft, G. (2001) Breaking bad news. *American Family Physician* 64(12), 1975–78.

Wallace, J. and Lemaire, J. (2007) On physician wellbeing—You'll get by with a little help from your friends. *Social Science & Medicine* 64(12), 2565–77.

Waldrop, D.P., and E.S. Rinfrette. (2009) Making the transition to hospice: exploring hospice professionals' perspectives. *Death Studies* 33(6): 557–80.

Walsh, K., Jones, L., Tookman, A., Mason, C., McLoughlin, J., Blizard, R. and King, M. (2007) Reducing emotional distress in people caring for patients receiving specialist palliative care. *British Journal of Psychiatry* 190(2), 142–7. DOI: 10.1192/bjp.bp.106.023960.

Walshe, C., Chew-Graham, C., Todd, C. and Caress, A. (2008) What influences referrals within community palliative care services? A qualitative case study. *Social Science & Medicine* 67(1), 137–46.

Waskul, D.D. and van der Riet, P. (2002), The abject embodiment of cancer patients: Dignity, selfhood, and the grotesque body. *Symbolic Interaction* 25(4), 487–513. DOI: 10.1525/si.2002.25.4.48.

Walter, T. (1999) *The Revival of Death.* London: Routledge.

Webster, R., Lacey, J. and Quine, S. (2007). Palliative care: A public health priority in developing countries. *Journal of Public Health Policy* 28(1), 28–39.

Whitaker, A. (2010) The body as existential midpoint: The aging and dying body of nursing home residents. *Journal of Aging Studies* 24(2), 96–104.

Bendelow, G., and Williams, S.J. (eds). (1998). *Emotions in Social Life: Critical Themes and Contemporary Issues.* London: Routledge.

Willmott, H. (2000). Death. So what? Sociology, sequestration and emancipation. *The Sociological Review* 48(4), 649–65.

Winter, L. and Parks, S. (2008) Family discord and proxy decision makers' end-of-life treatment decisions. *Journal of Palliative Medicine* 11(8) 1109–14.

Wittenberg-Lyles, E.M., Goldsmith, J., Sanchez-Reilly, S. and Ragan, S.L. (2008) Communicating a terminal prognosis in a palliative care setting: Deficiencies in current communication training protocols. *Social Science & Medicine* 66(11), 2356–65. DOI: 10.1016/j.socscimed.2008.01.042.

Witz, A. (2000) Whose body matters? Feminist sociology and the corporeal turn in sociology and feminism. *Body and Society* 6(2), 1–24.

Wong Y. and Tsai J (2007) Cultural models of shame and guilt. In J.L. Tracy, R.W. Robins, and J.P. Tangney (eds) *The Self-conscious Emotions: Theory and Research.* New York: Guilford Press, pp. 209–23.

WHO (2014) WHO Definition of Palliative Care. ttp://www.who.int/cancer/palliative/definition/en/

Wright, M., Wood, J., Lynch, T. and Clark, D. (2008) Mapping levels of palliative care development: A global view. *Journal of Pain and Symptom Management* 35(5), 469–85.

Zimmermann, C. (2007) Death denial: Obstacle or instrument for palliative care? An analysis of clinical literature. *Sociology of Health and Illness* 29(2), 297–314.

# Index

For Product Safety Concerns and Information please contact our EU
representative GPSR@taylorandfrancis.com
Taylor & Francis Verlag GmbH, Kaufingerstraße 24, 80331 München, Germany

www.ingramcontent.com/pod-product-compliance
Ingram Content Group UK Ltd.
Pitfield, Milton Keynes, MK11 3LW, UK
UKHW022125190926
475702UK00013B/1662

*9781138494855*